In the Arms of Angels

A Cancer Story

In the Arms of Angels

A CANCER STORY

STEPHANIE BOWEN

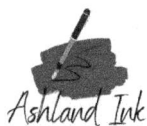

Ashland Ink

In the Arms of Angels
A Cancer Story
Copyright ©2025 by Stephanie Bowen
Book design copyright ©2025 by Ashland Ink Publishing

Author: Stephanie Bowen

Published by Ashland Ink Publishing
209 West 2nd Street #177
Fort Worth TX 76102
www.ashlandink.com

Published in the United States of America

ISBN: 978-1-963514-17-9 (paperback)
ISBN: 978-1-963514-18-6 (hardcover)
ISBN: 978-1-963514-19-3 (electronic book)

Dedication

I would like to dedicate this to my family. My mother was my primary caregiver during the darkest days of cancer. She would drive me to the beach so we could watch the waves and feel the healing energy of nature. Mom cried at night with me and laughed with me during the days to lighten my load. My sisters would provide food whenever I felt like eating, and watch countless movies with me to help bide the time.

My daughter Allison and husband Chris were my primary motivators to keep fighting and endure the treatments. They are my heart and soul.

And of course, to Dr. Hamid and the doctors at the Angeles Clinic. They never gave up on me. Without their tireless dedication to finding treatments for melanoma, I for one, would not be here.

Introduction

We all have a story. Our early childhood experiences shape our identity, along with other experiences throughout our lives - moments that leave indelible marks on our souls and direct our actions. Often, a significant event plays a pivotal role in defining who we become. This could be anything from a childhood divorce, a broken leg while trying to skateboard, a fall from a swing, or any emotionally charged moment that stands out in time. Strong emotional moments imprint themselves on your brain. That is why, at the end of their first week at school, a child, when asked what they learned, might recount an incident filled with emotion, like feeling upset when someone cut in front of them in the lunch line.

Each person experiences something that changes who they are and makes them the person they become. Like a plant provided with sunshine and water, we all grow as humans, our experiences feeding our souls. This is my story, one that took an unexpected turn and became life-changing not only for myself but for my entire family. We were deeply affected by a fight with stage four cancer, not knowing if I would make it through the insane concoction of drugs that did indeed keep me alive. Like the ancient marks of a raging river in limestone, leaving behind ripple marks indicating there was a water source in a now barren desert, my battle with cancer left its marks on me and my family. I am not alone in having this experience, as many people have fought cancer. And many people have not lived. This is my experience.

What defines a person? How do you navigate the world wanting others to see you? How do you see yourself? I had always seen myself as a teacher. Being an educator was my identity and passion for as long as I could remember. I started dreaming about this career at the age of eight. It truly felt like a calling, and I thought everyone around me also knew what they wanted "to be" when they grew up. I did become a teacher and was about halfway through my career when cancer interrupted my life. Then, cancer began a new identity.

Many people diagnosed with cancer refuse to let it define their identity. "You are not your cancer" can be heard in the cancer community. I am among a select few who have triumphed over a stage IV metastatic melanoma diagnosis. It is who I am. At the time of my diagnosis and treatment, there was a 5% chance I would live five years. Do I wish that I had not had to endure cancer? Of course, but that was over 12 years ago now, and I hold my head up high and own the experience. It is something to share to spread hope to others. Cancer does define who I am. My fight with stage four metastatic melanoma had me redefine my life's purpose, dive deep into myself, and create a reality and life mantra to be true to myself.

Being a mother, wife, and teacher ended. Moments like driving my daughter to her first dance or the bus stop and guiding her through middle school vanished. Heading to my school and greeting students, going home and doing chores - all over. Walking my sweet dog Abby in the snowy neighborhood we lived in - over. Once cancer is part of your reality, the solid ground beneath you is replaced by a fragile existence filled with doctor's appointments, hospital stays, scans, and countless needles that strip away your sense of humanity. You find yourself reduced to a mere shadow of who you once were, and there were many moments when I couldn't recognize myself.

My peaceful and isolated life in the high Sierra mountains was to be replaced by traffic jams on the 405 South into Santa Monica, California. Getting to the life-saving treatment would not happen immediately. It would take a few months for the correct diagnosis, and only then would the miracle happen that led me to the Angeles Clinic, where Dr. Omid Hamid saved my life. It would indeed take a miracle to save my life. Miracles and angels led me, and for reasons still unknown to me, I found the path to beating cancer.

Angels

Synchronicities are everywhere. That moment in your day when you don't feel like going on, but somehow you do. A stranger's smile, a green traffic light, or no lines at the grocery store when you're in a rush—these small moments accumulate. When coincidences happen repeatedly, they start to connect, transforming into something more meaningful than mere chance. Can you recall a moment when you were rushing because you misplaced your keys, only to arrive at your destination and discover a front-row parking space waiting for you? Or perhaps a time when you felt compelled to glance down a grocery store aisle and unexpectedly spotted a childhood friend? What if we began to view these occurrences as miracles? Many people envision miracles as grand events, like a cloud parting with angels singing. I believe that our angels accompany us in both the small and significant moments, and these moments add up to your life. Your life is a miracle, as I know mine is.

Every seemingly little detour and roadblock I

encountered while searching for a doctor to treat me contributed to the miraculous moments that ultimately saved my life. Throughout my cancer treatment. I was surrounded by miraculous moments. I chose to see the light and lean on my angels. If that led me to death, I was ready. Admittedly, it brought many tears, and I questioned whether my family was ready for me to die. Viewing my life path as a blessing and as something meant to be, helps me understand the purpose behind my cancer journey.

When you get cancer, you wonder why. Why me? It is a horrifying moment in your life to hear that you have a potentially life-ending disease without a cure. Though the reasons for my journey through this harrowing experience may forever elude me, I know I want to live and keep spreading the radiant gifts of HOPE and LOVE to all who grapple with the unfathomable diagnosis of late-stage cancer.

A belief in angels has always been with me, accompanied by an unwavering sense that something exists beyond death. Growing up in a non-traditional lifestyle with hippy parents, these beliefs were cultivated on their own, without the religious undertones of weekly church visits. My father was very anti-religious. His background as part of the Vietnam War generation, coupled with having a fervently religious mother, shaped him into a man who battled alcohol addiction and challenged societal norms throughout his life. My understanding of the afterlife developed organically as I read tales about near-death experiences and attentively absorbed the world around me.

My mother and father were quite young when twins came into their lives. I wasn't even part of their envisioned future! My mom was eight months pregnant, initially preparing for one child, when a doctor remarked, "You are pretty big, let's order an X-ray." That led to the surprising discovery of two babies. Twins... and then the challenge of choosing a second name. Stephanie. That's me—the unexpected second child of Linda and Randy Yates. I was even born second! Perhaps this unplanned existence fueled my desire to explore the concept of an afterlife, a thought I would contemplate endlessly during my cancer treatment.

As a young person, I began to embrace the idea of an afterlife after reading about near-death experiences. An author's account of leaving his body and coming back to Earth resonated deeply with me. Although I can no longer recall the title of that book, the notion that life extends beyond our physical forms stayed with me. It felt like a profound truth. Little did I know as a child that I would confront my own mortality at a young age in adulthood.

According to the National Center for Complementary and Integrative Health, a national agency within the National Institutes of Health, research indicates that music can significantly aid in healing. Music plays an important role in our overall health. It can relieve pain, reduce stress, and combat depression. It can be beneficial for a variety of health-related conditions. Research reveals that music serves as an aid for those in pain.

Music has played a vital role in my life since I was a child, with a favorite song always at hand and music constantly playing. Just one song can transport me to a completely different place.

Songs that mention angels have always resonated deeply within my heart and soul. From "Hark the Herald Angels Sing" to "Angel of the Morning" by Juice Newton, I was attracted to angels and any reference to them in music. The imagery of feathery wings and glowing halos captivated me. They symbolize innocence and support, leading me to envision angels surrounding us, offering daily support even when they are unseen. It was during my illness that I genuinely sensed their presence.

When I was young, as I sought to carve my own path in the world, attending college immediately seemed unattainable due to financial constraints. Instead, I took a summer job at Yosemite National Park. This experience only added to the sun damage my skin faced while I lay out by the Merced River in Yosemite Valley. I played "She Talks to Angels" by the Black Crowes on repeat. It was truly my 19-year-old self's anthem. I wanted to talk to angels.

This belief grew stronger throughout my cancer treatment, providing me with faith as I endured one of the harshest medical regimens designed to combat the black beast of melanoma as it spread like wildfire. I spoke with my angels. I needed to believe in something otherwordly because I didn't know if I would survive. I truly required angelic assistance to endure the painful treatments essential for my recovery.

Facing a diagnosis that required experimental treatments brought me into close contact with my guardian angels and numerous archangels. The instances that saved my life were more than mere coincidences. I will share more about that later. In short, I am truly a miracle.

...rest assistance to endure the painful period bears essential...
...a supervisor...

...tical... Moreover... required...national... this topic...
...might... exchange problems... more... challenged upon...
...timelines (phdmail). The results... that few doctoral students...
...on the... more... confidence... I will now... that... they...
...since it show... various... sufficient.

10

Diagnosis

*M*elanoma is a particularly aggressive form of cancer, known for its ferocity and fierce aggressiveness. With a high mortality rate, it's often difficult to overcome, especially when diagnosed at an advanced stage, which drastically shortens life expectancy. While it typically begins on the skin and can be curable if detected early, the real challenge lies in how it invades and spreads throughout the body.

Back in the fall of 2000, I had a small, early-stage melanoma. I was attending college at CSU Fresno when I noticed a tiny brown mark on the inside of my left forearm. It wasn't something that really stood out to me, other than being a bit itchy. My daughter (my first little angel) was a toddler at the time, and she pointed at it, saying, "Ouchie." That caught me off guard because it didn't hurt at all. I put a Band-Aid on it and just kept going about life. At the time, I was balancing finishing my bachelor's degree, taking teacher credential classes, and raising a toddler - there was no time for anything else. But when I noticed that the pigment from the spot was rubbing off onto the Band-Aid, I decided to head over to the University Health clinic to have the spot removed.

The first removal was a small punch biopsy. The doctor didn't seem overly concerned and removed the spot without much fuss. It did not take long for pathology to come back and inform us it was melanoma. At that time, melanomas were rated by how many millimeters into your skin the lesion went. Mine was classified as a Clark's level 4, which meant it had gone deeper than expected and required further investigation. The university doctor looked me in the eye and said she wanted me to be there for my daughter. Fear truly set in.

I was also required to do a sentinel node biopsy. This procedure involves removing lymph nodes that are closest to the melanoma. This procedure involves removing the lymph nodes closest to the melanoma to check if it has spread. They inject a radioactive fluid around the site of the melanoma, and then an X-ray identifies the nearby lymph nodes, which are removed for testing. If the melanoma has spread to the lymph system, it can move quickly to other parts of your body, making the situation much more serious.

A wide excision was also performed and then came the waiting game. Waiting for results is every cancer patient's worst nightmare. We wait, and we wait, and we WAIT! It completely robs you of your peace of mind as you sit waiting for the results. At the time, I didn't know it, but I would become all too familiar with this waiting game. When the results finally came back, it was good news. The melanoma had not spread to my lymph nodes. I was cleared, and life moved on. Annual skin checks and chest X-rays were required.

I moved forward with my dream job, teaching at a small, rural high school in Bear Valley, California. Living at 7,000 feet in the mountains was a dream. Surrounded by towering pine trees, vibrant lupine flowers in the summer, crystal-clear streams and lakes, and deep snow in the winter - it was a paradise. From our little historic cabin, I'd cross-country ski right to the front door of the quaint, ski-lodge-style school. On some days, after a big storm, I'd have to navigate through three to four feet of snow, summertime meant mountain biking right out into the forest.

There were few neighbors, but we were never alone. Bears, deer, raccoons, squirrels, and bluejays were always around, offering their own kind of company. Life in Bear Valley, California, fed the soul with a healing emerald nature. We were also far away from proper medical care. Far away from any cancer center.

I grew professionally as a teacher and worked very hard. I was a workaholic. My daughter grew up skiing and attending the same small mountain school where I worked. In my mind, I was convinced I had beaten melanoma. Ten years passed before it came back. It had been quietly lurking in the shadows, a tiny, microscopic cell somewhere in my body, just waiting. Waiting for my immune system to lower its guard. And when it came back, it hit like a wildfire.

By the time I was in my 30s, I began to feel invincible. After all, I had already beaten cancer once! I knew the dangers of melanoma. I knew it could come back. But once I hit the five-year mark after my stage one diagnosis, I began to feel like I had escaped its grip. I was even freer in the sun. There were countless times hiking in the beautiful forest, wearing just a small ball cap for sun protection. There might be a sunburn here and there, but nothing too serious. I took precautions, knowing the high elevation could be brutal on my skin, but I always thought I was lucky. Lucky that I'd caught it early.

Another factor that contributed to the cancer returning was something quiet and insidious - stress. Constant exposure to stress weakens the immune system, making it harder for the body to fight off illness. The immune system needs to be at its best to battle things like viruses and cancer cells. According to the National Library of Medicine: "In contrast, long-term stress suppresses or dysregulates innate and adaptive immune responses by altering the Type 1-Type cytokine balance, inducing low-grade chronic inflammation, and suppressing numbers, trafficking, and function of immunoprotective cells." In layman's terms, the more stress you endure, the less equipped your body is to fend off cancer cells.

My life wasn't the idyllic, utopian existence it might have appeared to be. Teaching was becoming increasingly more stressful, and I was under constant scrutiny and criticism from the community members in Bear Valley. My goal had been to gain acceptance in this small town, but the harder I tried, the more I felt like an outsider. Everyone wants to feel supported, to feel like a part of a community. But no matter how hard I worked at it, I always felt like I didn't quite fit in, and that just added to the mounting stress. The workaholic tendencies I'd developed began to take a serious toll on my family, creating turmoil at home.

My personal life was becoming increasingly unsettled. My husband and I went through a long stretch of disagreements about everything—how to live, what to prioritize, and where we were heading. We found ourselves arguing constantly. He started spending more and more time away from me and the cabin. The possibility of divorce or separation was even brought up. This was especially hard on our young daughter. The stress was building, but I didn't realize that I was working myself into a grave. Our bodies aren't meant to be in constant "fight or flight" mode. That kind of relentless stress creates the perfect breeding ground for a weakened immune system. And in that weakened state, cancer would find a way to resurface, and this time, it wouldn't be the small, eraser-sized freckle I'd once had but something much more dangerous.

Somehow, I had lost my way. I thought I could force things to happen—work hard enough for community respect and provide a stable home for my daughter so she wouldn't experience the kind of unsettled life of homelessness I had known. My vision, though unrealistic, and my ego led me to believe that as a teacher, I really mattered to my community. But in reality, I didn't. I fought every day for professional respect and hoped for the recognition that never came. Instead, there was constant criticism. To make matters worse, I was a control freak, trying to influence everything and everyone around me. This kind of lifestyle wasn't sustainable; it created a Petri dish of stress. Controlling everything would simply lead to almost losing everything. In the process, my body became the perfect breeding ground for illness. One of those little malignant cells was melanoma. Once it was let out, it was a hurricane.

The Fight Begins

The year 2010 started like any other. I turned 40 and still worked too much. My daughter started middle school, and unbeknownst to me, she was becoming the target of severe bullying. On the surface, it seemed like we were living the dream, nestled in the mountains, surrounded by skiing, hiking, mountain biking, and swimming in crystal-clear lakes and rivers. We loved everything about our environment. But beneath it all, something was deeply out of balance.

Life requires balance, a trifecta of three essential elements. Those include your home life and the relationships that exist there, your environment, and your professional life. When these three things are in balance, you can absorb stress. For example, if you have a loving, supportive family and a job you're passionate about, but your city or neighborhood doesn't resonate with you, your spirit can balance this out. You can absorb the stress. But when more than one of these elements is out of balance, it causes stress and you become unstable. No single part of your life's trifecta can carry the weight on its own and maintain your mental and physical well-being. Imagine a tripod. If one leg is shaky, the other two absorb the instability. But if two legs are unstable, the whole thing collapses. Life's trifecta demands balance to survive and thrive.

I lived in a beautiful environment that I loved. Tall pines, blue skies, flowers, crystal snow fields, and high Sierra lakes surrounded us. My work life was a mess. I worked 9 to 11-hour days and was under constant scrutiny. Criticism from the community was relentless, and parents were never happy with our school. My personal life was not healthy, and my husband and I were barely speaking to one another. My workaholic habits were putting immeasurable stress on my marriage. Two crucial elements of my trifecta were completely out of whack and unstable.

Living this way is unstainable. Over the years, the constant strain took a huge toll on my heart and soul. It was an extremely dangerous way to live, especially for someone with a history of cancer. Constant small illnesses plagued me. Bronchitis was a "normal" part of life, along with other viruses. My patience for even the smallest inconveniences had worn thin. I remember actually having a mental breakdown over something trivial one day and crying and crying uncontrollably heading home from work. I would pay for this imbalance dearly and almost lose my life over it.

Around April of 2010, I discovered a small pea-sized

lump in my left armpit. Or did I? When you're busy, it's easy to overlook such things. Staying busy was my specialty. Avoiding "things" that were upsetting had become a skill! In May, I felt something again. Is it bigger? " No," I told myself. Ignoring it some more became my coping mechanism. I was too busy, and I felt the weight of responsibility on my shoulders, or did I put it there? As the primary breadwinner for my family, I had a young daughter to raise. I was finally a teacher and was desperately trying to prove my strength and worth to my small community while struggling to fit in. I did not have time for cancer. It was easier to ignore symptoms.

Deep in my left armpit, it floated. At times, I would feel it, while other times, it seemed to vanish. Deep inside, I was worried. I knew it could be something bad. October arrived, marking breast cancer awareness month and prompting more self-exams and a mammogram following a check-up in September.

Then came September 2010 - there was no denying it anymore. There most definitely was a lump. It could no longer be ignored. I had to face the reality that something malignant was developing.

School had started, so I had plenty of distractions. My latest teaching assignment was not easy. After ten years of teaching high school ELA and Social Studies, my beloved little Bear Valley High School was closed down, and I was transferred into the elementary education side of the school. Rumors quickly made their way to me that people did not trust me and did not understand why I had been given a position in the elementary school. Pressure to gain acceptance weighed heavily on my heart. I was tasked with teaching third, fourth, and fifth grades, with only one student in each grade level. Teaching in this small mountain town was both a dream come true and a source of great stress. The community was highly critical of everything happening within the school, and staff constantly felt the need to appease parents, yet it never seemed to be enough. The stress was overwhelming. Combined with an overbearing administrator, I was an unbearable ball of stress and ready to burst, like an infected splinter that needed to be released from the skin.

By now, we had lived in Bear Valley for ten years. I found that my workaholic tendencies widened the massive gap between my husband and me. In a town that felt unwelcoming, work was all I had to cling to. Chronic stress can indeed be a ticking time bomb within your body.

Before I faced the mystery lump, I was dealing with a plantar's wart that served as a troubling distraction. I truly believe this was a precursor to getting cancer. Located on my left foot, the same side as the cancer, it was situated beneath my big toe on the ball of my foot. It hurt like hell, and after trying to treat it myself, I ended up in the podiatrist's office to have it carved out of my foot. This landed me on crutches. The chronic illnesses I was facing were taking their toll!

Not long after this experience, the lump under my arm

began to reveal itself as the monster it was destined to become.

Something frightening was happening in my body as a growth was taking root under my left armpit. I would later learn it was wrapping around my brachial plexus nerve. With every millimeter it grew, the pain intensified. Squeezing and squeezing, tighter and tighter. It felt as if a spider was gradually encircling my left shoulder, tightening its grip relentlessly, and it seemed impossible to escape without undergoing one of the most toxic treatment regimens in the world.

Around Halloween of 2010, I found myself back at my primary care doctor's office following my mammogram. I mentioned that I felt something in my left armpit. After examining me, she confirmed that there was indeed something she hadn't detected just a month earlier. My heart dropped as she ordered an ultrasound and referred me to a surgeon.

Oh, shit! Things were getting real.

The ultrasound yielded no definitive results. But something was there. I knew it! I could feel this lump that was now a small marble. My new doctor, a general surgeon, ordered a CT scan. As Thanksgiving drew near, the lump continued to grow. Determined to maintain control and avoid troubling anyone, I drove alone to Mark Twain Hospital in San Andreas, California, for the scan. I wanted to spare my family from worry. Inside, however, I was gripped by fear, feeling as if I were detached from my own body. Emotionally, it was an out-of-body experience.

I recall walking into the CT scan room and putting the gown on. I lay down, stretching my arms above my head. This marked the beginning of many scans that would soon become a routine part of my life. My heart raced, and I felt an unsettling intuition that something was bad. Deep down, I feared that the melanoma had returned, but I was too scared to admit it. As I got dressed again, the technician reentered the room. Normally, results take time, and we had grown accustomed to hearing, "See you next Monday." However, the technician nervously mentioned what the radiologist had observed. It's generally not the role of radiology techs to share this kind of information. "The doctor thinks the cancer is back."

What the actual hell? *WHAT THE HELL??!!* I froze. The dressing room walls felt like they were closing in on me. This was really happening. How do you cope with cancer when you live in an isolated mountain town at 7,000 feet elevation and the closest cancer center is over an hour away? How do you tell your family? How would I tell my adolescent daughter? A whirlwind of terrifying thoughts flooded my brain. I knew it was over. My life was over. How would I make the most of my final days? I truly believed I was going to die. At that moment, I found myself alone with more than an hour's drive ahead of me. Terror gripped me, especially knowing that melanoma is deadly. Once it spreads internally it's nearly always fatal.

The First Time

In the fall of 2000, while I was still a student at CSU Fresno, melanoma first appeared in my life. At 30 years old, I was completing my teaching credential and raising my sweet daughter.

My daily routine involved taking Allison to the preschool campus at Fresno State at 7:30 a.m. After dropping her off, I would drive across town on Highway 41 to downtown Fresno for my student teaching assignment at one of the city's most underprivileged schools. After a day filled with teaching and learning, I would hurriedly return to the preschool to pick up Allison. We would then head home for dinner. Once Allison was settled and asleep, I would dive into my homework. This routine continued for several months.

The cancer first appeared as a very small spot, as small as the head of an eraser. Just an innocent-looking little freckle. No worries, nothing to see here. I was trying to ignore it. But it was itchy. One day, my baby pointed to it and said,

"Ouchy!" For some reason, I put a Band-Aid over it. When I took it off, the dark color had rubbed off onto the Band-Aid. At that moment, something inside me knew it wasn't right. But I was too caught up in everything else to think it could be something serious.

My family persuaded me to have it removed, leading me to the university health clinic. With graduation just a year away and while I was in the process of obtaining my teaching credential, the timing couldn't have been worse. But, if you ask any cancer patient, they will share that they also had no time for cancer. No one has time for cancer.

The biopsy results came back, and that dark spot turned out to be melanoma. It would require a sentinel node biopsy and a wide excision of the surrounding tissues.

A sentinel node biopsy is used to determine if the cancer has left the primary location and spread to neighboring lymph nodes. Your lymph system is a filter for your body. As you exercise, lactic acid develops in your muscles. This filters through the lymph system. If you get small injuries on your skin, the lymphatic system helps heal you. Mosquito bites? The lymph system helps. But, it can also be a roadway for cancer cells. Once cancer cells enter your lymph system, they can easily spread.

This procedure was relatively simple compared to what lay ahead when the melanoma came back. They begin by injecting a radioactive substance around the original melanoma site and then take an X-ray. The sentinel nodes light up and are marked with a Sharpie. Oddly enough, there was no anesthesia for this procedure, and I remember the nurse telling their assistant, "Hold her arm so she doesn't hit me." It struck me how some medical professionals have such vastly different bedside manners. In the end, three lymph nodes were marked for removal.

I vaguely remember the procedure. I was praying so hard that the cancer was not in my lymph system. At that time, the only thing I knew about melanoma was that it killed people. The procedure was done at the Veterans Hospital in Fresno. We didn't have health insurance, so I ended up at the same hospital that treated inmates. Having a specialist never even crossed my mind.

What crossed my mind was, "How will I ever enjoy being in the sunshine again? How will I do the things I love the most because all of these things are outside in nature?" As soon as I wrapped up my education, we were leaving Fresno and heading to the mountains. We wanted to raise Allison in the forest, skiing, hiking, and camping. I did not have time for this bullshit!

During this stage of my life, my experience as a patient was limited to two instances: 1) giving birth to Allison and 2) breaking my leg in my twenties due to a skiing accident. Undergoing a surgical procedure felt entirely new to me, and I was nervous. I wanted to be there for my family.

After the surgery, I returned home and bought a lot of long-sleeved shirts. I vowed never to sunbathe ever again. Waiting for results is absolutely agonizing. Everything slows down, and you jump every time the phone rings (yes, landlines). This was before everyone had the internet at home, and luckily, I did not have Google at my fingertips. Nonetheless, I knew that melanoma was a death sentence.

In an effort to stay upbeat and not get too depressed, I entered a local radio station contest and made up a song about the surgery and the possibility of cancer. I won! My story and song were so depressing and real. I don't even know what I won, but it was likely a lunch at Subway.

A few days later, the call arrived. The cancer had not metastasized. It was not in my sentinel nodes!

At last, the moment had come to ride off into the sunset and live my life footloose and fancy-free. I hugged my family and put on my long-sleeved shirts. My follow-up appointment at the health clinic left me bewildered as now my doctor was telling me not to overreact.

Ironically, she stressed the importance of being there for my daughter. I refused to let this close call prevent me from truly living! I plunged back into my everyday life with renewed energy, resolute in my decision not to look back.

Doctors

It's important to take a moment to reflect on the role of doctors, and how my perception of them evolved over time, especially during my battle with cancer. When a doctor enters the room in a white coat, many of us instantly see someone we believe to be extremely intelligent. And often, that's true. Earning a medical doctorate is no small feat—it's a deep commitment to helping others, and doctors hold a lot of power in their hands. But we must also remember that doctors are people too. They operate with the best knowledge they have at any given moment, but that knowledge is still limited and always evolving.

Doctors come in different tiers. There are those at the top of their field, like Dr. Omid Hamid at the Angeles Clinic, who not only excels in treating patients but is also pioneering treatments for melanoma. Then, there are those whose expertise might be more focused on diagnosing common conditions like bronchitis or pneumonia. The distinction between these types of doctors is important to recognize. They are not all the same.

The surgeon at the veteran's hospital who called me with the news that the cancer hadn't spread was still learning, but I could feel his genuine empathy and concern on the phone call. On the other hand, the doctor at the university health clinic was probably not someone who should have been dealing with melanoma in a patient. Then there was the general surgeon, a specialist in hernias, who should have never continued seeing me when the cancer came back ten years later. His failure to properly evaluate the growing lump in my left armpit could have killed me. I am amazed I survived being his patient.

To say it is imperative to see a specialist is an understatement. In most medical fields, and especially when it comes to cancer, there are so many subcategories that only experts in those areas truly know how to navigate. Patients really need to take charge of their own future and be advocates for themselves.

Patients should always attend a doctor's appointment with someone else. Take notes, and write down your questions. If you don't feel a connection with your doctor, seek a second opinion. We must always do what is best for ourselves. If your doctor's ego is too big and they walk in swooshing their white coat and stethoscope, acting as if they know it all, dismissing you... run! If they are not a specialist, go to a specialist. If you think you have cancer, go to an oncologist, for crying out loud!

Right now, I find myself reflecting back to November

2010. This is when reality came slamming down on me. The reality was that the melanoma had returned, which meant this could be my final Thanksgiving and Christmas. I was under the care of a general surgeon who continued to advise me to return the following Monday. For fuck's sake.

Stage 4

*A*s I drove home from the Mark Twain Hospital in San Andreas, having been told that the cancer was probably back, my thoughts were consumed by Allison, who was just 12 years old. Being a mother was my most important job. I truly wanted my daughter to have a better life than I did. I knew that my parents did their best, but I didn't want Allison to endure the hardships of homelessness or grow up amidst alcoholics and addicts. I wanted her to have a strong, solid home where she felt safe. Now I had to tell her I was sick. At this time, I did not know what she was experiencing at school.

After spending six years at our small mountain school in Bear Valley, my daughter transitioned to a new middle school. I aimed to allow her to experience a larger school environment and integrate with a new group of peers before high school. This plan backfired, as she quickly became a victim of bullying. My happy girl, who loved hiking, skiing, and the mountains, quickly transformed into a sullen, dark, and sad individual. Self-harm started to emerge. I had no experience in parenting a young girl, and I constantly pestered her to open up to me. Allison began to struggle with depression, and shortly after, I was diagnosed with late-stage cancer. Sadness only intensified when I had to leave in search of medical care for my cancer. The awesome life I thought I had built for our family in Bear Valley was falling apart.

Navigating adolescence is challenging enough. During this time, you seek acceptance and strive to make a good impression on your peers. Allison was already burdened by the sadness stemming from the marital problems my husband and I endured. When the cancer diagnosis was added to her already fragile state, it plunged her into a deep spiral of sadness and depression, from which she would require years to recover.

When I told Allison I had to leave for cancer treatment, it was the saddest moment I had ever experienced. Breaking the news to my dear daughter was truly heartbreaking, and I felt as though I was abandoning her. During this challenging time, Allison entered a dark period, reaching out to online friends who may not have been truthful about their identities, all while facing one of the harshest winters Bear Valley had seen in years.

We lived at an elevation of 7,000 feet, where winters brought approximately 30 to 50 feet of snow. Our cabin became snowbound, necessitating a snowmobile, cross-country skis, winter boots, or snowshoes for access. The winter of 2010-2011 was particularly challenging, as it brought an extraordinary snowfall exceeding 50 feet while I fought cancer. This massive snowfall often resulted in power and phone lines being down.

Despite being advised against it, Allison couldn't help but search online for information about melanoma and soon realized that this was extremely serious. Her father worked night shifts, hoping that Allison would be asleep, but instead, she filled her mind with upsetting information. During my treatment, heavy snowstorms would bury our small cabin. Allison persevered as her father took on the roles of both dad and mom. I had to completely let go and leave. My life depended on it. I couldn't just sit in the cabin and die. I was in desperate need of a miracle, as the cancer was spreading rapidly. I was a very sick person with absolutely no idea where to go. How in the world do you get yourself into a cancer center?

Even with the news I received, I had an annual trip to Yosemite planned for the next month. My mind was numb to the severity of the situation, and since I figured I was dying, I was determined to go on this trip.

The third weekend of November has traditionally marked the annual Serenity in Yosemite AA/Al-Anon conference. Since my father struggled with alcoholism, I attended Al-Anon, which led me to participate in the Serenity in Yosemite conference for many years.

Although I had a large tumor growing in my left armpit, I went to Yosemite with my husband, daughter, and mother.

We slept in tent cabins. I could feel the tumor growing every day. It was a perplexing time since I had not yet received an official diagnosis, and the new doctor was attempting to identify the issue through a needle biopsy. I was trying to maintain a "normal" life amidst all the appointments. My mother was frequently present, and my sisters were aware that I was dealing with a potentially life-threatening illness, yet I still had not received an official diagnosis!

As we attended the meetings and discussions at the conference, I found myself reflecting on what I believed would be my final visit to one of my favorite places. I vaguely recall feeling as though I were going to die. My fighting spirit had not yet been ignited. That weekend, snow blanketed the area, with large snowballs crashing down from the trees, sounding like bombs striking our tents. Fear consumed me, completely distracting my attention. The needle biopsy had failed to provide a diagnosis. Surgery to remove the tumor was scheduled at Mark Twain Hospital in San Andreas, under the care of a general surgeon, just before Thanksgiving. My confusion and lack of information about my health and what was starting to kill me would prove to be almost fatal.

On December 9th, 2010, my calendar read, "shit hit the fan." "It's malignant," the doctor said. It was melanoma, stage four. It had returned, and it was terrifying. The medical professionals looked at me with pity. I did not want to be one of those who had a "meaningful experience from cancer." What the hell was I going to do?

The beginning of my treatment was incredibly frightening. The pain was overwhelming, and I was consuming large quantities of Vicodin. It felt like time stood still. I had walked through a door, and I could never return to the life I had known before. That was not an option. It was time to warrior up and fight for my life.

Rewind, How Did I Get Here?

*W*hat events in my life contributed to being diagnosed with melanoma, the deadliest form of skin cancer? How did I get here? Naturally, many cancer patients ponder their journey and what led to their diagnosis. For a lifelong smoker, a lung cancer diagnosis might not come as a surprise. Similarly, a person who loves candy and sweets probably won't be surprised by a diabetes diagnosis. Likewise, individuals with a genetic predisposition to breast cancer are often prepared for such news. However, many melanoma patients are unaware of the origin of their primary tumor. In my case, the cause was obvious.

Growing up in Laguna Beach, California, bikinis were the quintessential accessory for all girls. It was typical to own several bikinis and spend an excessive amount of time sunbathing. It was common to go to the beach right after school and lay out in the sun. A tan symbolized health and wealth. People even tanned during ski trips to Tahoe! Whether surfing or playing beach volleyball, everyone tanned. If you were concerned about too much sun exposure, you simply applied SPF 4 Tropicana. A typical summer involved wearing your swimsuit from sunrise to sunset throughout the season. From Memorial Day weekend to Labor Day, all the kids in Laguna wandered about in swimsuits. It was perfectly normal to aim for the darkest tan possible, surrounded by chocolate-brown bodies from childhood into young adulthood.

We had no idea that just one blistering sunburn could increase our risk of melanoma by 50%. We were unaware that at least three of our classmates, myself included, would battle this disease, and one of us is no longer with us. We also didn't know that some of us would lose family members to melanoma. This reality was simply unknown. Our goal was to be bikini babes. The boys were surfers, and we girls were beach babes. Salty, tanned skin, which often meant a constant sunburn, was our way of life in Southern California.

In the carefree days of the 80s, as I blasted Duran Duran, Bon Jovi, and Oingo Boingo on my Sony Walkman, I unknowingly set the stage for skin damage and created the perfect environment for cancer to thrive. My part-time job at a tanning salon likely added to the problem. Sadly, many young people resort to tanning beds to achieve that "healthy glow" for spring breaks, proms, and other occasions. This belief that tanning is beneficial has resulted in numerous young people, especially young women, harming their skin and developing melanoma. While I may never know if this was a contributing factor to my situation, it's certainly a strong possibility.

If I could travel back in time and advise my 16-year-old self to cover up, I'm certain that young Stephanie would dismiss any warnings, as teenagers are inherently stubborn and willful. They feel invincible, and I was no exception.

Leaving the Mountains

When reality hit and I knew it was in fact cancer, it was time to flee to a place that would save my life. Staying in the mountains would only mean death. After Thanksgiving in 2010, we knew it was time to take action. By that point, I had already undergone surgery to "remove" the tumor. My mother and husband accompanied me to San Andreas for the procedure.

After the surgery, the doctor emerged from the operating room to meet my family in the waiting area, looking as pale as a ghost. What he found inside of me was not something he could remove. This doctor was, without a doubt, the wrong choice for my surgery, and his attempt to excise the tumor could have potentially cost me my life. He had no business doing this, and I am lucky to be alive. This marked the beginning of a difficult period, enduring two JP drains protruding from my left armpit, inserted into the bloody mass of a melanoma tumor he encountered when he opened me up to "remove it." I won't mention his name, as this was a botched procedure that should never have occurred. I learned that doctors are practicing medicine, and it's crucial to verify their credentials before allowing them to operate on you. We often place doctors on pedestals, but that is not where they belong.

Perhaps it is unfair to place high expectations on someone solely based on their title as a doctor and their white coat. Are we demanding too much from a mere human being?

During one of my last appointments with the general surgeon in San Andreas, I overheard the doctor instructing the nurse to administer a pneumonia shot, as I was likely going to undergo chemotherapy. This was mentioned as if I were not even present, as a side note before he washed his hands of me. I will never understand why that doctor continued to see me for so many weeks. I do not understand why he hesitated to refer me to an oncologist immediately. It was truly absurd that he kept attempting to manage the tumor himself. It was equally ridiculous that I did not see the writing on the wall - that I was sick! Finally, when the test results confirmed it was malignant, I was referred to an oncologist in Lodi, California.

In Lodi, I had my first PET scan. I remember feeling incredibly sick. Everything around me was hazy, and the pain was intense, radiating from my left armpit throughout my entire body. What I didn't know at the time was that the cancer was beginning to spread. Perhaps the attempt to remove the tumor had released cancer cells into my bloodstream. After a surreal afternoon of being scanned in a mobile scan trailer, we finally made our way to the oncologist's office. It was late in the day, and my mom, my husband Chris, and I sat in a cold, unfriendly office. The doctor was more than 40 minutes late. When he finally walked in, he casually said, "I could have done this over the phone." Chris turned white. The doctor's words were chilling: "Go home and get your affairs in order."

That was the moment when my true battle commenced. Inside, I was so angry at myself and the doctors. At that moment, the anger fueled me, and I knew it was time to fight. Anger can be a powerful motivator. Reality smacked me, and I was ready to fight.

As we began our drive up into the mountains, our first stop was to pick up Allison. Our daughter had been in the care of good friends in a small town approximately 40 minutes west of Bear Valley. I cursed the entire drive home. Anger continued to motivate me. I desperately needed to find someone who could save my life—a specialist or, at the very least, a cancer center far removed from the small rural towns where I was seeking assistance. To say we were all in shock would be an understatement.

This marked the beginning of the journey of being a cancer patient. We gathered my young daughter, Allison, and drove up into the mountains through a white-out blizzard. After our snowmobile ride back, I had to share the devastating news with Allison. Even 13 years later, that moment still breaks my heart. Telling my daughter that I was seriously ill was far more painful than the illness itself. No child should have to face the possibility of losing a parent. My mom and I began reaching out to everyone we knew, calling upon the universe for help. We had no idea what to do; we just knew we needed help. Gaining access to a reputable cancer center without a doctor's referral is challenging, especially with the holidays approaching quickly. We contacted numerous places across California, from UC Irvine to Hoag Cancer Center in Newport Beach. Securing an appointment felt impossible, and with the tumor continuing to grow, time was running out. It was truly a matter of life or death.

This is when you start to transition your life into patient mode. It was during this time that I discovered the importance of being my own best advocate and realized that a supportive team was essential. My team consisted of my family: my husband, my mother, my twin sister, and my younger sister.

We called cancer centers, doctors - anyone who might be able to help. I was desperate, past the point of feeling like I had control, but I knew this was my life. That asshole in Lodi wasn't going to tell me to just get my affairs in order. I packed a bag, still on Vicodin, with the two JP drains hanging from me, and I said goodbye to my family in the snowy parking lot of Bear Valley, my beloved little mountain town.

It broke my heart to say goodbye to my family. Allison's face filled with disbelief and terror as she faced growing up without her mom. Chris, too, felt a part of himself fall into a pit of despair as I drove away. Suddenly, he was a single parent, facing the terrifying possibility of losing his wife. For a moment, he even pondered returning to his old demon of alcohol, but he knew Allison needed him.

Angels began to help! The little moments that led to much-needed help began to accumulate. My mom and I traveled to Sonora, California, to retrieve my tissue samples, knowing they would be essential for the journey ahead. However, we were still uncertain where we were going. We only knew we had to leave. We raced toward Southern California, where my parents lived. It's difficult to recall the emotions we experienced during this time. My mother, Linda, suddenly had to transition into a full-time caregiver for her adult daughter, while I had to relinquish my adulthood and independence. We felt lost in both time and space, facing a future that felt like the darkest night, with no moonlight to guide us and no sign of dawn to assure us that life would go on. How does one prepare for the possibility of death at 40?

The next part of this story serves as proof that angels are real. Angels exist all around us. They are more than mere heavenly beings floating around. The next series of events began the road to healing and beating cancer. But, I was acutely aware that my chances of survival were uncertain. Deep down, I knew I was dying.

As we journeyed south through the golden hills near Merced, California, a random phone call came in from Carla, the spouse of a long-time friend who lived in New York. Her husband was one of my best friends. Angelic assistance from people I did not know began to come through in waves. Suddenly, there was a glimmer of hope, and I reached out to it like a lifeline in an angry ocean. Carla mentioned she "knew someone who knew someone" on the Board for the Melanoma Research Alliance named Debra Black. The Melanoma Research Alliance (MRA) was established following Debra Black's stage II diagnosis and has become one of the leading funders of melanoma research globally. Debra was acquainted with Dr. Donald Morton at the John Wayne Cancer Institute in Santa Monica, California. Both were involved in the MRA, where Dr. Morton developed the sentinel node lymph biopsy procedure. Tragically, he passed away in January 2014. Dr. Morton served as the chief of the melanoma program and co-director of the surgical oncology fellowship program at the John Wayne Cancer Institute, earning a reputation as one of the best melanoma surgeons in the country. Securing an appointment with him just a week before Christmas without a referral was a miracle.

With Carla's help and the virtual introduction to Debra Black, we managed to schedule the appointment during the hectic holiday season. This wasn't a guarantee, and I was still dealing with the pain from the JP drains. The discomfort was intense, and I was heavily relying on Vicodin. We made the long drive south, stopping in Bakersfield to visit my kind-hearted in-laws, Aunt Barbara and Uncle Alan, at their home, which they affectionately called "Helton's Hilton." They are some of the sweetest people. They had no idea just how sick I was. They didn't know that I had a 16 cm tumor growing under my shirt.

As devoted members of the Church of Jesus Christ of Latter-day Saints, my uncle and a fellow church member gave me a blessing for healing. They laid hands on my head and prayed. It didn't matter to me that I wasn't a member of their faith. What mattered was the energy of the prayer, and the sense of healing it brought became essential to my survival. I didn't follow a specific religion, but I welcomed all prayers. I simply believe in a higher power watching over us, along with the presence of guardian angels. During my journey as a full-time cancer patient, I received prayers from many, from strangers in a thrift store to those at a post office. Mindful prayers filled my heart constantly as I fought cancer. Prayers for strength to say goodbye were especially important if that became necessary for my daughter.

My physical health had begun to deteriorate significantly. My body was fighting malignant melanoma, a black beast. And the cancer was winning. The pain was both unbearable and relentless, leaving me debilitated. All I could do was manage day by day, hour by hour, as I waited for the appointment with Dr. Morton at the John Wayne Cancer Center.

At that moment, I began to realize the truth that I was deathly ill. I had cancer. There was no mystery about my condition. Cancer was spreading and growing within me, and I was suffering. As Christmas approached, I genuinely felt like this might be my last Christmas. I was no longer a mother, wife, or teacher. I was now a patient who would become accustomed to wearing hospital gowns, being poked and prodded, and being looked at with sad faces because I looked like death, bald and skinny. I needed to become knowledgeable about all things cancer-related. My husband and daughter were on their own. I had truly hoped to protect Allison from the horrors, but leaving our mountain home would only cause her extreme stress and sadness. My husband, too, would suffer as he contemplated a future without me and questioned the purpose of his ten years of sobriety. Everything was different, and not for the better.

It is difficult to comprehend and explain what cancer does to a family. When the cancer diagnosis hits, a family is thrown into chaos. Suddenly, you're forced to understand the ins and outs of health insurance—what it covers, and what it doesn't. You have to become fluent in medical jargon just to navigate the system. And all the while, you're trying not to cry, because your loved one might die.

The business of cancer for our family was indeed left to my husband. Chris was the one facing bill after bill, each one larger and more overwhelming than the last, all for treatments that were supposed to save my life. The financial strain was unfathomable, and the emotional toll was just as heavy. On top of that, he was buried under a mountain of snow from massive winter storms and even deeper in the avalanche of medical bills that seemed impossible to pay. At one point, my insurance kicked in 100%, and a healthcare nurse from the insurance company was assigned to advise me on making healthy choices in my diet. I figured they had spent so much money on me that they wanted to make sure I lived. Meanwhile, the little medical coverage I had through my school district was quickly maxed out, overwhelmed by the astronomical costs of my care.

My first visit to John Wayne Cancer Center involved a series of extensive tests, including a brain MRI, a PET/CT scan with contrast, and blood work. At this time, my pain levels were still quite high, and I felt an overwhelming sense of fear. I had never undergone a brain MRI. The process was quite daunting as I was slid into the large, spinning cylinder, accompanied by a constant thumping sound. My head was secured in a small, cage-like device, requiring me to stay perfectly still. Additionally, I had to drink a CT contrast solution for the first time, with mocha or mixed berry flavors added to make the barium sulfate beverage somewhat more enjoyable. Yuck!

Following the tests, I found myself in the office of Dr. Donald Morton on December 22, 2010. Accompanying him was a resident attending doctor. Dr. Morton, who introduced himself as the top melanoma surgeon in the county, always had a resident by his side, resembling someone straight out of central casting. After all, we were in LA!

The exam began with him requesting my consent for a physical check-up, and I removed my gown. The presence of two JP drains surprised the doctors. While examining the large tumor, Dr. Morton listened to my story about how I arrived at his office. He asked if I had experienced any stressful events. Chris and I exchanged glances, fully aware of the strain our marital separation had placed on our family and my work. We were open about everything. A surgery was scheduled for January 5, 2011, to remove the tumor. It was also time for me to get accustomed to undergoing scans. Throughout my treatment, I would undergo numerous PET scans, CT scans, and brain MRIs.

Mom and Chris accompanied me to the imaging department of the hospital, where I was admitted for a PET scan. This procedure involves injecting a radioactive fluid and then lying still for approximately 50 minutes. The radioactive material is absorbed by any cancerous lesions, allowing the metabolic rate to be measured. The more a lesion metabolizes the radioactive sugar solution, the stronger the indication of cancer. My PET scan showed significant activity. Fortunately, a brain MRI indicated that the cancer had not spread to my brain.

We were all still in shock as we drove back to Orange County to celebrate Christmas to the best of our ability. Keeping hope alive was difficult, but we were making progress, and a qualified individual was helping me!

It was nearly Christmas Eve, and we were all focused on making the best of things for Allison. Then, at 7:00 p.m. on

December 22, 2010, the phone call arrived with the test results.

There would be no surgery. The cancer had spread, now affecting my lungs and causing subcutaneous lesions to appear. I was completely lost and devastated. Silence spread through our awkward Christmas celebrations, marking one of the most devastating moments for my family. I am certain that the large doses of Vicodin contributed to my spiraling mental state. We were all in shock, unsure of how this would unfold. My husband, daughter, and I cherished each moment together, believing this might be the last Christmas I spent with Allison. It truly felt as if my heart were breaking.

After Christmas, Chris and Allison packed up our little Subaru and made the eight-hour drive back to Bear Valley, leaving me behind to stay and receive the life-saving treatment I needed. As they headed into a brutal blizzard, it felt like our small, tight-knit family of three was being torn apart. The hugs were not enough to ease my mind that Allison would be ok without me. Little did we know, this would plunge her into a dark place that would take years to recover from. The goodbyes didn't bring me any comfort. There's no way to say goodbye to your child, knowing it could be the last time you hold them and not feel completely devastated. But even amidst the extreme sadness, I knew it was time to dig in and fight against this bastard cancer that had started to take over my life.

Dr. Morton arranged an appointment for me at the

Angeles Clinic on January 2, 2011. This meant enduring the agony of my advancing cancer in the meantime. There were countless moments when I should have gone to the ER for pain relief, yet I remained in bed, overwhelmed by pain and a deep sadness that felt like a hole in my heart. I missed my daughter immensely. All I could do was wait for the upcoming doctor's appointment, hoping it wouldn't be too late.

2011

$\mathcal{A}$ new year began, and my twin sister and my mother drove me to Santa Monica. The journey along I-405 north from Orange County to Los Angeles would soon become a familiar route. Upon arriving at the Angeles Clinic, we were struck by the welcoming atmosphere and the healing energy radiating from the sleek professionals walking the halls. Sheek, clean, and, at that time, relatively small, the environment was inviting. Everyone greeted us with genuine kindness and warm smiles. Despite the shared burden of facing the daunting diagnosis of a deadly cancer, we were all treated with utmost dignity. Located in a city known for its glamour and fame, here we were naive about the treatment ahead and how difficult it would be.

Upon our arrival, we were warmly welcomed by the receptionist, Maria, whom my family would soon know very well. We were then escorted to a standard exam room, where I changed into a cloth gown while Mom and Kathryn took a seat. Shortly after, a tall and handsome doctor,

Dr. Omid Hamid, entered the room alongside Maggie, the oncology nurse assigned to my case. Unbeknownst to us at the time, he was a prominent leader in melanoma research, actively involved in the development of ipilimumab, a precursor to many FDA-approved drugs today. He proceeded to examine the area around the JP drains, as well as the sizable tumor.

After reviewing my physical condition and the scans from my December visit with Dr. Morton, he told me I was an ideal candidate for biochemotherapy. Dr. Hamid, with his gentle yet straightforward approach, reassured me that if "the shit hit the fan," he'd let me know—but, thankfully, it wasn't time for that just yet. His honesty, combined with kindness and compassion, immediately gave me a sense of hope.

He also noticed I had been on Vicodin for weeks and was struggling with severe constipation. He prescribed something for relief, and I was soon given a shot in my buttock, which was the first time in weeks that I felt any kind of comfort. Dr. Hamid explained that I would begin biochemotherapy in just three days. There was paperwork to handle, and a port would need to be put in, but this was the first real step forward.

For the first time in weeks, I thought I might live. A light was beginning to shine, and it was coming from the Angeles Clinic. "Ángeles" is the Spanish word for "angels," and it means to be in an angelic state. Angels were definitely present.

The time spent waiting between my initial appointment and entering the hospital was extremely challenging. The pain overwhelmed me, leaving me in a hazy state where I felt detached from my body. I practiced deep breathing and counted the minutes until I could return to the hospital for stronger medication through an IV. My spirit was truly being tested as I lay in my parents' bed (my father moved to the daybed in the living room), staring at the ceiling and praying for relief. During these moments, I sensed a presence holding me. A presence of warmth and love assured me that no matter the outcome, whether it be life or death, I would be OK. I knew that someone was watching over me.

I attempted to Google biochemotherapy, but since it's such a rare and intense treatment, I could only locate one other individual who had undergone it. It truly was a last-resort option, and even now, I am aware of only two other people who have been prescribed this extreme therapy.

On January 6, 2011, I arrived at the hospital at 6:00 a.m. for my port surgery, which would mark the beginning of my treatment that same day. At that moment, I hurt everywhere. Pain rippled through my body. Every movement intensified the discomfort, especially as the stiff wheels of the wheelchair rolled across the hospital's laminated floors. Simple tasks became a struggle, and I could no longer maintain the facade of being a strong patient. I yearned for immediate relief, but I would have to endure much more before the pain subsided. Reflecting back to 1992, when Chris and I obtained our marriage license, I remember the requirement of a blood test, which terrified me due to my fear of needles. My fear of needles has been erased by cancer treatment. I would soon become a human pin cushion with a double access port that would allow medication to be delivered into a large vein near my right collarbone.

The biochemotherapy treatment required a five-day hospital stay at the start of a 22-day cycle. I would check into the oncology ward, where the regimen was an intense combination of three chemotherapy drugs and two immunotherapy drugs, all administered together in a fierce assault on the rapidly spreading cancer. It was going to be brutal.

The plan was an IV push of vinblastine, nine oral chemo pills of temozolomide, and cisplatin via an IV drip over two hours. Along with those, I'd have a constant drip of IL-2 for the full five days, and every night, a shot of interferon. We dubbed the interferon "shake and bake" because of the wild side effects it caused. The handout detailing potential side effects was a daunting 15 pages long, listing a laundry list of symptoms I had never even imagined.

Possible side effects included, but weren't limited to, blood in my urine, vomiting, diarrhea, dizziness, loss of balance, hearing issues, shortness of breath, fever and chills, sore throat, seizures, changes in urination, rapid heart rate, itching, uncontrollable nausea, black tarry stools, confusion, irritability, depression, and yellowing of the skin and eyes.

The treatment was designed to make me feel like death itself.

Walking even five feet to the bathroom would be almost impossible, and a simple ride in a wheelchair would make me dizzy like I had motion sickness. I wouldn't be able to eat for days. I would lose all my hair. And there would be so many tears, though I tried to cry alone so I wouldn't drag anyone else down.

But in the middle of all that suffering, I would dig deep inside, trying to find the faith that I could survive this. Faith that some power greater than myself could provide a sense of sanity in the darkest days.

The initial treatment felt like a blur. Following the early surgery to insert the double port, I was placed in a room on the fourth floor, the oncology unit. I was relieved to receive stronger medication than Vicodin for the pain and grateful to be under general anesthesia. A few hours after the surgery, the treatment began.

I remember asking a nurse if my hair would fall out. I received anti-nausea medication through my IV, while one access point of the port provided a steady flow of hydration. Ativan became a regular part of my routine. Soon after, the IL-2 (interleukin) drip would start. Following that, I underwent chemotherapy treatments, with a daily interferon shot given around 6 p.m. It's hard to fathom receiving such a high dosage of cancer-fighting drugs for a typically drug-resistant cancer like melanoma. Patients who were only treated with IL-2 often needed to be admitted to the ICU due to its toxicity.

Biochemotherapy has since been replaced by newer treatments developed at the Angeles Clinic. Looking back, this type of treatment seems like the worst possible approach for treating cancer. But, stage four melanoma required the most extreme attack humanly possible. The odds were stacked against me. Back then, the survival rate for stage IV melanoma was grim—just a 5% chance of making it five years.

Calling All Angels

The drive from Laguna Woods to Santa Monica on I-405 is a short distance, but because of traffic, it became a long one. "Calling All Angels" by Train played as we made our weekly trip to the hospital. Even today, this song brings tears to my eyes. We waited in endless lines of cars, trucks, and buses, watching the millions of people living their busy, normal lives in Los Angeles - people running errands, going to work, seemingly existing in a reality that did not include cancer. As we drove at a snail's pace, crawling by LAX and creeping closer to Wilshire Boulevard my stomach began to churn just knowing what was coming.

At the time, my mom had a VW Passat with heated seats, and those seats saved my ass, literally. The chemo had started to trigger arthritic symptoms in my hips, and the heat was the only thing that could offer any relief. I'd sit in the passenger seat, tears streaming down my face, feeling the weight of it all, too weak to drive, too weak to care for myself. A simple five-foot walk to the bathroom toilet was all I could muster. The phone call I had to make was like I was checking into a luxury spa in LA, but really, it was to the oncology ward, telling them I was on my way to start yet another round of treatment.

Instead of massages and facials, I was reminding the nurses about my port placement, asking them to use a 1 ½ inch needle because my port was slightly deeper under the skin. After circling the block to find street parking, we'd drag ourselves to the front doors of St. John's Hospital, and then it was up to the elevator. I'd be assigned a room, and soon, the medicine would begin to flow into my veins.

Hospital stays were surreal. My mother or sister always stayed with me, ensuring I would never be alone. I insisted that they take breaks during the day to get some fresh air. Kathryn would usually head to the local Whole Foods, hoping to spot a movie star. They'd sleep on the tiny bench in the window of the room. We tried to pass the time by watching the movies they provided, though I lost track of how many times we ended up watching "Salt" with Angelina Jolie. My chemo brain could never fully piece together the plot. Was she a Russian spy or really American? Meals were brought to me, but the nausea took over every time, and I'd ask my family to take the food away. I simply couldn't eat.

During that time, my mental state was tenuous. The fragility of my life screamed that every day could be my last. As I began treatments, I made a decision. First, I was not going to die. Second, if I died, I would do it with dignity. I would be a model patient and take my medicine with courage and dignity. On the outside, I kept a smile on my face, polite and courteous to those around me. I discovered that this helped my overall well-being. When I was alone, in the late nights or in the early mornings, I would let the tears flow down my pillow. Sobbing, I would let the warm, angelic energy flow into my spirit, filling me with just enough strength to face one more day. One more day of opening my eyes and seeing the skyline of downtown Los Angeles, silently hoping that this wouldn't be the last view I'd ever have.

At my parents' home, where I was now living, I had taken over half of their bedroom and half of their king-sized bed in their one-bedroom apartment. Mom and I shared the bed while Dad slept on the daybed in the living room. But there were nights when he'd leave the house to sleep in "Homie"—his 1978 Dodge RV parked in a lot nearby. Dad didn't handle this well. Watching his daughter fight for her life interrupted his lifestyle. His alcoholism was still very much alive, and so was he until an alcohol-related health condition finally took his life in the form of a massive heart attack.

It was here, in my parents' bed, that I felt death. In those early weeks, the pain was so overwhelming that I clung to deep breathing and the belief that angels were taking care of me. From my research of Doreen Virtue's teachings, I came to sense their presence. It was both a relief and scary to realize that any night could be my last, but despite that, I kept opening my eyes each morning to face the cancer.

I remember one particular moment just before treatment when I felt the presence of my two guardian angels. I prayed that they would take away my unbearable pain. As I lay in my parents' bed, with my family far away, a profound loneliness washed over me. I knew, deep down, that these could be my last days. I knew it. In my heart of hearts, I felt as though I were floating away, dying. I felt the presence of my angels. They were right behind me, and it felt like my life ended. Their glow comforted me. Death didn't claim me that night. With each deep breath and every prayer, I made it through. I truly believed I was going to die, yet my body was fighting to live. Somehow, through it all, I woke up the next morning - and I was still here.

Simply getting an appointment with a doctor right before Christmas felt like a miracle. But to end up in the office of the doctor who had pioneered sentinel lymph node biopsies? That felt like fate. And then, to find myself at the Angeles Clinic... Angeles, which means "angels" in Spanish! I had to believe. My daughter needed a mother. And I was facing the most toxic cancer treatment in existence.

As the cancer treatment began, I dug in for the battle. I gave up on balancing a checkbook, deciding what to make for dinner, or planning lessons for my classroom. I was now 100% patient Steph, with my family fully committed as Team Steph. They vowed to never, ever leave me alone— someone was always by my side, in my hospital room, throughout every treatment. Mom, Kathryn, or Chris would take turns, each staying with me through one cycle. They'd sleep on the small window bench in my hospital room. They watched as each medication was administered. We ended up watching the same movies over and over again.

Archangel Raphael represents healing, and he's often associated with the color green. During my first cycle of biochemotherapy, something extraordinary happened. A CNA walked into my room, and his name tag read Rafael. He radiated love and care in a way that filled both my mom and me with hope. He had the face of an angel. Rafael was incredibly handsome, and his eyes sparkled. The unknown was terrifying. His aura settled and calmed us during those first moments of treatment. Many nurses came and went after him, but we never saw Rafael again. I honestly believe he was an angel appearing at exactly the right moment to bring us the reassurance we so desperately needed. His energy felt like a miracle, a brief, perfect moment of calm when we were overwhelmed by the monumental task of the treatments ahead.

After returning to my parents' apartment following the first treatment cycle, we found a pendant in my mom's parking garage, one with the image of Archangel Raphael. I knew, deep in my heart, that this was a real sign that angels had my back. I was not alone. And even if I died, they would take care of my family.

The treatment continued. It started with that first call to the hospital to check in, then taking the anti-nausea meds to prepare my body for what was coming. Nurses would hook up my port to the chemical IV tree, which would administer the drugs. Most people picture an infusion center for cancer treatment with comfy recliners and soft lighting, but my treatment had to be done in the hospital because this particular regimen was so intense that it could kill me if I were not carefully monitored. Nurses and doctors checked my vitals every four hours. Often, they'd struggle to get my blood pressure and would have me shake my legs.

The treatment days were dark. Often, I took the maximum dose of Ativan just to get through. The pain from so many drugs was unbearable, and I didn't know how I'd make it through the treatments. The first cycle shocked my body, and I was sicker than I'd ever been. I vomited frequently and descended into a chemically-induced mental haze that lasted for months. My focus and memory were compromised. By the second cycle, my hair started falling out, and I had to cut it. I was losing weight. When I started treatment, I weighed about 175 pounds, and by the end, I was down to 122 pounds. Cycle three was pure torture, and I had many mental breakdowns. I didn't think I could continue the treatment. It seemed impossible. Side effects took over. I had severe rectal bleeding, probably from the immunotherapy, and my sister shaved my head as more clumps of hair came out.

One day, my mom and sister went to a pharmacy near the hospital to pick up my pain medication. I was taking about 80 mg of OxyContin. When they tried to get the prescription filled, the pharmacy assistant treated them like criminals. All they knew was that I needed pain relief. Unfortunately, I needed a lot—around 80 to 100 mg a day of opiates. That was the only thing that helped numb the pain.

Soon, I looked like the scary kind of cancer patient that made people look away. I was an old woman, barely moving, barely alive. During treatment, I stopped wanting to be awake. I just accepted whatever medicine that would put me to sleep. Tired of the pain from cancer on my left side and from the port on my right side, I just wanted to sleep through it all. I no longer ate. I couldn't even hold a pen when I was asked to sign the advanced directive. Surprisingly, I never signed it. I saw it as admitting defeat. Even in my darkest, most confused moments, I wouldn't allow cancer to win. Even if I was going to die, I wanted to go out fighting.

What do you say to someone who is dying?

During one checkup with Dr. Hamid after treatment, he asked if I was feeling depressed and when I had last eaten. I had barely eaten—just half a cup of applesauce in almost ten days. Food was impossible as the nausea never stopped. If I ever felt hungry, it was usually around the 20th day of the 22-day cycle, right before heading back to the hospital. After the fourth cycle, I was so broken that I cried through my entire appointment, begging to be done. Dr. Hamid didn't want to stop the treatment because it was working. He agreed to give me an extra five days before starting the fifth cycle, and for the first time, I began to feel a faint stir of hunger. At one point, I was offered the chance to join a clinical trial for ipilimumab, which would eventually become the FDA-approved treatment Yervoy. The paperwork was confusing, and I couldn't fathom starting over again. I had been through so much already, and because I was one of the rare few for whom biochemotherapy was actually working, the thought of beginning a new treatment felt unbearable.

Back in 2011, during my treatment, I didn't have the support from other melanoma survivors that I have now. It was a lonely place to be. It felt like everyone and everything from my old life had forgotten about me, and all I could focus on were hospital beds and surviving each day. By the middle of treatment, I was taking around 80 mg of oxycodone a day for the pain. Chemotherapy had started to take its toll on my motor skills, and my brain was showing the effects, too. I struggled to stay focused, my thoughts feeling scattered. I updated people through CaringBridge, though, and tried to remain positive in my posts, even though I knew my cognitive abilities were compromised. Here are some of those entries, left unfiltered, a reflection of where I was at the time.

The CaringBridge entries capture a time when I truly felt close to death. The treatment was brutal, and few people can endure receiving four chemo drugs and two immunotherapy drugs at once. I tried with everything I had to remain "positive," but that is nearly impossible when you're trapped in that kind of headspace. Like a flower waiting in the Sahara Desert, waiting for rain to finally fall and quench its endless thirst, I waited for the medicine to do its thing and for the cancer to stop growing. This was when I developed a patience I never knew I had, as each treatment cycle took away Stephanie, the teacher, mom, and wife, and replaced her with Stephanie, the cancer patient. These entries are unedited, reflecting the rapid decline of my mental state and the growing difficulty I had focusing. At one point, I figured I wanted to die as a positive patient, the one whom nurses remembered as kind. I would die with dignity.

Friday, December 3, 2010, 9:26
Today is okay... I am waiting for Monday, but trying to stay in the moment. Monday is my first surgery. I start with a small one, to remove part of this mass in my armpit. I am glad to get rid of some of it. As it is very uncomfortable. Thanks for the love.

Saturday, December 4, 2010, 7:05 a.m.
Went to visit my students yesterday. It was good to see their little faces! They made cards for me. One little guy loves ninjas and drew some for me. It was good to see them and my school. I miss it!

Monday, December 6, 2010, 12:06 p.m.
Hello Everyone, This is Kathryn, Stephanie's twin sister reporting on her behalf. She is out of surgery. It was pretty extensive and she will return to Dr.next week. We are still waiting for a concrete diagnosis. Thanks everyone for the prayers.

Tuesday, December 7, 2010
Hi everyone, The biopsy was rougher than I imagined, but Chris & my mom are taking care of me. Once the general anesthesia wore off, by this morning, I definitely felt better. The doctor told us he was able to get a decent sample for the pathologist who was on site at the hospital. I am resting and healing from the procedure. Please understand if I do not answer the phone. I am pretty tied and on some painkillers so I am a little loopy. Thanks for the love!

Thursday, December 9, 2010, 7:55 a.m.
Good morning, I feel okay today, getting ready to make BIG decisions about my health. I want to share that my official diagnosis has NOT come in yet. We are awaiting the official report from the pathologist. I am grateful for all the well wishes from everyone and appreciate it more than you all know@@ Monday is a post-op appointment and I will know more.

Sunday, December 12, 201010:45 a.m.
Tomorrow I get this drain out of my arm, getting sick of it, and is very achy... & we get the results from the biopsy.

Monday, December 13, 2010
Today I heard what I knew was coming, but I do not think it was easy for anyone to hear. It is melanoma in my body. Luckily, it appears to not have spread to my organs. Tomorrow I meet an oncologist who can provide more info about my condition. Too surreal for words.

There are no CaringBridge entries for the oncology visit in Lodie, CA. That was the visit that I was told to go home, he could have done the visit over the phone, and to get my affairs in order. That was when I declared war on Cancer. Even though I had NO idea of where I was going.

Thursday, December 16, 2010
I am out of the mountains and seeing a cancer doctor at UC Irvine who specializes in melanoma. Keep praying! Thanks, LOVE Steph

Thanks for all the prayers and love, It's working. A special thanks to Spencer and Carla in New York for the connection. I will do a post-surgery when I can. Merry Christmas.

Friday, December 17, 2010, 10:58 a.m.
I have an appointment to see one of the BEST melanoma doctors in the country at the John Wayne Cancer Institute, Dr. Morton. Thanks to my dear friends in New York for networking with me. Much love to you across the country!! Feeling hopeful, loving this battle is not an option.

Saturday, December 18, 2010, 5:18 p.m.
People are inquiring about my mental state and I wanted to say I think I am doing pretty well. I have expressed sadness with crying, and anger with some special words, but anyone who knows me knows I wear my heart on my sleeve. What you see you is what you get thus no poker games for me. Anyhow, I am doing well. I feel as though the right thing will happen for me and my family. Take Care of yourselves and Merry Christmas to everyone!

Thursday, December 23, 2010
Dear Family and Friends,
Hello to all, this is Kathryn, Steph's sister reporting on her behalf. This morning Stephanie saw Dr. Morton at the John Wayne Cancer Center in Santa Monica. She is currently going through a battery of tests, CAT scan, PET scan, MRI, etc... She is going in for surgery on January 4th, 2011, and will follow up with radiation treatment. The doctors are wonderful according to Steph and Chris. She is in really great spirits and said everyone is being really nice to her. (as they should).

Friday, December 24, 2010, 6:53 p.m.
Dear Family and Friends, This is Kathryn again with an update on Stephanie. Apparently, the doctors have changed their plan of attack on Steph's cancer. They want to do chemotherapy first to shrink the tumor and then do surgery. Things changed quickly. Thanks for the prayers. Keep on praying.

Monday, December 27, 2010, 10:22 a.m.
It is Monday and I am waiting to see a medical oncologist. More waiting...(Big SIGH) I think everyone is on vacation for Christmas but cancer does not take a holiday. This is very frustrating and I am becoming an expert on waiting. Happy New Year Everyone...

Tuesday, December 28, 2010, 10:15
I am still waiting for the medical oncologist to call me. The plan for now is to receive biochemo before the surgery as the tumor is very large and with sadness, I share that the cancer has spread to the lungs. I read about others who have gone through stage IV melanoma and survived and the doctor has never indicated that my situation is hopeless. It will be extremely tough when it starts but I am too stubborn to give up. Anyone who knows me will agree that I do not give up easily. I am very sad but doing my best to stay strong.

Wednesday, December 29, 2010, 10:23 a.m.
My next stop is the Angeles Clinic in Santa Monica to see Dr. Hamid. His bio is great, he sounds brilliant and kind. I see him Monday, Jan 3rd. Thanks for all the wonderful messages.

Tuesday, January 4, 2011
Dear Family and Friends,
Kathryn here with an update. Yesterday we went to the Angeles Clinic and saw Dr. Hamid. He was amazingly kind to Steph. After an initial exam, he found another tumor on her abdomen. At some point, he looked her in the eyes and told her he would save her life and she would be a survivor. We got new pain medication for her and are going back to Brentwood today to finish the paperwork. He wants to admit her ASAP to start biochemotherapy. She will be hospitalized (hopefully by this Friday) for 5 days, then out for 2 ½ weeks then hospitalized again for 5 days of treatment. After a 21-day cycle her cancer will be restaged via CAT scans, PET scans, etc. The side effects are serious but she is young and healthy despite the cancer.. I will update again when she is admitted to the hospital. It is St. John's Medical Center in Santa Monica, Take Care all.

71

Behind closed doors, a team of doctors was reviewing my case. Led by Dr. Omid Hamid, they reviewed my information. By the time they got involved, I was gravely ill. My chances of surviving five years were just 5%. These doctors were some of the brightest minds in the field of melanoma, people who had committed their lives to finding a cure. They used precise calculations and strategies to treat each patient who entered the Angeles Clinic.

Here are some of the notes from my treatment, and looking at them now, it's horrifying to realize just how fast and aggressively the cancer had spread. The medical team knew how difficult it would be to stop. At the time, I didn't fully understand that the cancer had already reached my bones. I was so sick and in so much pain that simply surviving the treatments was all I could focus on. Survival was my only thought.

The medical notes were in the hands of the people trying to save my life. I'll never know exactly what was said in those meetings. But I imagine, based on the treatment I received, that those conversations were full of both intelligence and compassion. These weren't just doctors trying to find a cure for cancer—they were people trying to cure me. They were trying to give me back to my family. I envisioned them around a table, like knights gathered at the Round Table, not planning to slay dragons, but to figure out how to save my life. These warriors were fighting for me. The following comes from those meetings...

Medical Notes: Metastatic Melanoma

Patient Names: Stephanie Bowen

DOB 3-1-1970

CT CAP RIM

Clinical History: Melanoma: mass left axilla

Comparison: ETCT 11/20/2010

Chest CT: Findings: A large left axillary mass is increased significantly in size in the interval measured at 9.6 x 8. versus 7.6 x 6.0 on the previous exam. The lesions are likely engulfed by a few additional smaller adjacent nodules present on the prior exam at the inferior aspect of the mass. A catheter has been placed in the interval with the distant portion of the mass (left lateral percutaneous chest wall approach.)

There are new pulmonary nodules present as follows: 10 x 13 mm right lower lobe nodule, image 41; 12 x 11 mm lower left nodule, image 42, lobulated or two cluster lesions at the left perihelia region at the border between lover lobe nodule and upper lobs measured at 19 x 16 mm, image 27 and stable ovoid within the right upper lobe measured at 11 x 5 mm and likely represents a benign process.

Conclusions:
- **Rapidly enlarging dominant mass at the left axilla. A catheter entering from the left lateral chest wall area is noted with its distal portion curled within the mass.**
- **New pulmonary nodules consistent with metastases.**
Abdomen CT

Findings: A few hypodensities within the liver are consistent with cysts. The liver is otherwise normal in size, density, and enhancement pattern without suspicious mass or dilated ducts. A new 15 x 13 subcutaneous nodule present at the anterior abdominal region, image 39.

The spleen, kidneys, adrenal glands, pancreas, and gallbladder are normal. There are no enlarged lymph nodes, ascites, or suspicious bone lesions identified.

Conclusions:
- New subcutaneous 15 mm at the anterior abdominal wall consistent with metastasis.

These findings were from tests that were done before I found my way to Southern California. The next set of results were from the John Wayne Cancer Center.

Name: Stephanie Bowen
DOS: 12/23/2010
Pet / CT Skull to midthigh
Clinical History: Melanoma; mass left axilla
Conclusion:
- Rapid increase in size of intensely hypermetabolic left axillary mass.
- New hypermetabolic pulmonary nodules and solitary subcutaneous anterior abdominal wall metastases.
- New and enlarging bone metastases.

Exam: MRI Brain WO & W contrast on December 23, 2010, 11:43 AM

AXILLA: : Technique: The following images were obtained in a high field MRI scanner: There is no hemorrhage, mass lesions, midline shift or fracture. No evidence of acute ischemia. The orbits and paranasal sinuses are grossly unremarkable. No abnormal enhancement. The skull base, cavernous sinus, calvarias, and IAC are grossly unremarkable. Impression: No evidence of metastatic disease in the brain.

Exam: Nuc Bone image study
Service date: 01/07/11
Procedure: after intravenous administration of 33 mCi of Tc99MDP, whole body views were obtained after an appropriate delay.

Findings: Symmetrical tracer uptake is observed throughout the skeletal images, including symmetrical increase at the shoulder and hip joints. There is a single isolated focal increase at the costochondral margin of right anterior rib #6.

Here is asymmetry of the soft tissues, appearing significantly more abundant associated with the left chest and axillary regoing. Physiologic bilateral renal function is incidentally noted.

Impression:

1. Arthritic-appearing reaction at shoulder and hip joints.

2. Probable mild traumatic or inflammatory reaction at the right anterior 6th rib.

3. Asymmetry of left chest and axillary region soft tissue. Correlation is recommended.

DOS 02/14/2011
PET SKULL TO MID THIGH
DOB 03/11/1970
Referring Physician Dr. Omid Hamid
Clinical History: Melanoma
Procedure: Multi-station, co=registered PET/CT images of the body were obtained from the skull base to the pubic cubmyhis using Siemens Sensation 16 biography PET-CT Fusion scanner following the intravenous injection of 12.2 mCi of FDG, glucose 109.

Findings:
Neck: No abnormal accumulation of radionuclide is present.
Chest: There is a 5.2 x 6.2 necrotic lesion within the left axilla with peripheral rim hypermetabolic activity and SUV 4.4.
Abdomen / Pelvis: No abnormal accumulation of radionuclide is present.
Conclusion: Hyper metabolic left axillary lesion with significant central necrosis measuring 5.2 x 6.2 cm. No other lesions are present.
These test results indicate that the treatment is working!
DOS: 02/14/2011
CT Neck /Chest/ABD/PELW/ w/wo contrast
Technique: CT scan of neck chest, abdomen, and pelvis with and without contrast was performed on the Biemens Biograph CT/Pet fusion scanner with contiguous 5 mm asixal images obtained from the skull base through the pubis symphssis. The patient was examined both and following the uncomplicated IV administration of 100 mL of Ultravist 300.
CHESt: The Lungs are clear without evidence of focal opacification, effusion, phneumothorax, edema, or nodules. No pulmonary mass lesion or metastases are present.

By mid-February, I was well into my treatments. My only goal was to survive. It was physically demanding, and I'm not sure how I endured it. The biochemotherapy required me to go to the Angeles Clinic after each hospital stay for hydration, and I'd get a shot to boost my white blood cell count. My family and I would stay at the local Best Western. The drive to the hospital felt like hell. The one block to get there seemed like miles, and I could barely make it to the room without throwing up. Once, I had so much rectal bleeding that we were all really scared. The immunotherapy caused a huge rash, and I spent a lot of time lying in a shallow bathtub trying to cope with the painful side effects. It was crucial to stay nearby since I couldn't handle the long drive back to my parents' apartment.

At the Angeles Clinic, they monitored me and checked my overall health, but honestly, I don't remember much because of all the medications I was on. At one point, they asked if I was depressed. Uh, yes! They also asked how much I'd eaten. About half a cup of applesauce in two weeks. My weight dropped from 175 to 130 pounds. All my hair fell out, and scarves became part of my daily routine. Everything hurt. I didn't even know if it was worth it - the constant pain, the injections that felt like glass shards in my veins. My once healthy, hiking body was being reduced to a bald, frail version of itself, with skin hanging off my bones.

DOS: 03/28/2011
PET - Skull to MID THIGH
Comparison: 02/14/2011
Procedure: Multi-station, co-registered Pet/CT images of the body were obtained from the skull apex to the pubic symphysis sing the Siemens 16 Biograph Pet-CT Fusion Scanner following the intravenous injection of 12.6 mci of FDG. Glucose 110.

Findings:
Head / Neck No abnormal accumulation is present.
Chest: Minimally increased radionuclide activity is present at the periphery of low density 5.1 x 4.5 cm left axillary mass with an SUV of 2.7, previously 5.2 x 6.2 and SUV 4.4

Abdomen:/Pelvis: No abnormal accumulation of radionuclide is present.
Skeletal: No abnormal accumulation of radionuclide is present.
Normal physiologic activity is present in the brain, heart, liver, gastrointestinal tract, and genitourinary tract.
Conclusion: decreasing in SUV minimally hypermetabolic necrotic appealing left auxiliary mass.

By this point in my treatment, I had completely broken down. While I smiled on the outside, my insides were beat. At night, when I was alone, I cried. That's when I allowed the tears to roll down my cheeks. On top of dealing with the 15 pages of side effects from the treatment, I was also suddenly thrust into menopause.

At 40, my ovaries died. My pillows were soaked with sweat, and there was a long period of bleeding at the start of treatment, but then it stopped. In the years that followed, I would only have about four or five more menstrual cycles. Going into full menopause at 40 made my internal parts feel like those of a 70-year-old, and this led to lifelong issues that took me years to understand and deal with. Experiencing this normal biological event so young created confusion. I didn't realize the full impact until about seven years after surviving. That's when I started reflecting on my symptoms and understood the truth: internally, I was at least 20 years older than my actual age. I felt like a raisin left out in the sun too long. My personal and intimate life suffered because of it, and I needed answers. This was just one more thing that cancer did to me. This bastard disease tried so hard to take everything, and I fought just as hard against it.

My heart was shattered because I couldn't be there for my 13-year-old daughter, Allison, as she navigated middle school. She was experiencing some of the toughest emotional times of her life, and it would take her years to recover. Depression led to self-harm and thoughts of suicide. With the massive winter storm in Bear Valley, the phone lines were down for days, and there were no cell towers, so I couldn't even hear her voice. To say I was devastated doesn't even cover it. A hole had been ripped in my heart, and all I wanted was to go home. But I couldn't. I had to stay and keep facing the treatments because if I didn't, the cancer would win. It was working, and I had no other choice.

Allison's life was never the same after cancer. She had been the happiest little girl, always the one to approach other lonely kids, offering a smile and a helping hand. But while she waited at home in our cabin, her sweet, kind soul seemed to fade into sadness and despair. She was told not to Google anything about the cancer, but no one was there to stop her. Soon after, nightmares started to plague her sleep, dreams of wildfires or tsunamis coming to destroy everything. Even now, 14 years later, she still struggles with restless, nightmare-filled sleep. It took years before she started to heal.

I just wanted out of the hospital rooms and clinics. I was a mess, completely drained from the constant pain, the poking to access my port, the fluids, and the chemicals being pumped into me to monitor the cancer. After one incident, where a tiny nurse was literally on top of my chest, trying to get a needle into my port, I realized I needed to tell the medical staff that I needed a longer needle. My port was at an angle under my skin, and they hadn't been using the right size.

I walked into my doctor's appointment in March and just broke down, crying. I wanted to quit. I couldn't see how any of this was worth it anymore. Death would have been welcome to end the suffering. Now, that may sound a bit dramatic, but I truly was at the bottom of a dark pit, and looking up, I could no longer see the light. It was exhausting to be "positive" and "happy." If you ever hear someone say they can't take any more treatment, know that it's not just physical exhaustion—it's the pain of being so disconnected from your life. Mentally, there's only so much a person can handle. Dr. Hamid told me he'd give me an extra week between cycles to help me recover. The treatment was working, and his goal was to get me through six cycles of biochemotherapy, six 22-day cycles that were saving my life, but also absolutely brutal.

Relying on my angels became a bigger part of my life as time went on. I wasn't exactly sure who they were, but I always felt the presence of two beings close by, especially during the two times I truly thought I was going to die.

One time was at my parents' house before treatment started. I lay in bed in more pain than I had ever experienced. Closing my eyes, I prayed that there would be a solution. There was a warm and glowing feeling behind me. All I had to do was breathe deeply, sink into myself, and it would be ok. The next thing I knew, I opened my eyes and was still alive. This would be an experience that materialized many times.

Another time was in the hospital room at St. John's during a treatment cycle when I was barely conscious. Nurses and doctors were in and out, checking my vitals every four hours. At one point, the nurse asked me to sit up and shake my legs, saying, "Honey, I can't get your blood pressure." My heart kept beating. My eyes would open, and I'd see the skyline of downtown Los Angeles, and for a moment, I thought that might be the last thing I ever saw. Seriously? The last thing I'd see would be LA? People should be able to die where they want to, surrounded by the things they love. Dying in a hospital isn't anyone's choice. Dying at home, with familiar things and the view out the front window, is what most would prefer. Unfortunately, many don't get that choice. And because I chose to fight, I was in a hospital. The fourth floor of St. John's Hospital in Santa Monica, California - this is where I might expire.

When the medical part of the treatment ended, there was surgery. The tumor, still inside me, was no longer active. It was a dead mass. The huge 16 cm tumor had stopped showing up in PET scans, but after seeing Dr. Morton, we decided the next step would be to remove it. He recommended doing a complete dissection of all the lymph nodes in my left armpit. Dr. Morton agreed that the surgery was necessary to take out the dead tumor, the surrounding tissue, and test everything to make sure the cancer was truly gone. I had to wait four weeks after my last treatment to allow my body to heal enough to be strong enough for surgery. My heart felt heavy because that meant I couldn't go home yet. I was so homesick, longing to be with Allison and Chris in our mountain cabin. By now, I had received 25 doses of interferon, which I didn't know at the time, but it caused depression. I was definitely feeling a deep sadness, missing my daughter with my entire being.

Surgery was scheduled for late spring 2011. I remember the morning we woke up to go to the hospital. Of all the memories I have from that time, one stands out: I thought I could actually eat this time. During all my previous hospital stays, I was so nauseous that I couldn't eat anything. I had to have all the food taken out of my room immediately. Food just didn't happen. But this time, I could wake up from surgery and eat. It's strange what our brains remember.

This hospital check-in felt different from all the others. I arrived at pre-op and weighed in at 125 pounds. I had started treatment at 175 pounds. I was skinny and weak, but also feeling a deep sense of gratitude for making it this far. I lay in the bed as doctors and nurses prepped me. By then, I was a professional patient, used to needles, IVs, weigh-ins, and blood pressure checks. In my hospital gown, I was rolled into the operating room. The anesthesiologist gave the classic countdown, and then I was out. The next thing I remember was waking up in post-op, which, for me, was on the oncology ward.

Phew, I had made it through another milestone. To my surprise, they had placed a catheter so I could rest more comfortably. And despite thinking I'd finally be able to eat, I was served a diet of jello and broth.

After surgery, my family met with Dr. Morton, the sweaty and exhausted surgeon. He was the best melanoma surgeon at the time, and he explained how carefully he had to remove the dead tumor wrapped around my brachial plexus nerve. It was a long, complicated, and delicate procedure. The cancer had been tangled up with sensitive nerves, and preserving the use of my arm required incredible precision and attention to detail. To this day, I'm convinced that Dr. Morton is the reason I can still use my left arm. My husband had thought I would come out of surgery with no use of it at all.

The waiting game continued. Waiting to leave the hospital, waiting to heal, and waiting for the test results on the tissue and lymph nodes that had been removed. They placed another JP drain in my left armpit. When the post-op visit came, I had no idea what I was going to hear. Had all those months in a hospital bed actually killed the cancer? Melanoma was known for being resistant to treatment.

Relief flooded over us as my family and I realized there was no evidence of cancer anywhere. The surgery had been the final step of my active cancer treatment. I was a miracle.

This was an angelic moment. Relief washed over me, and I felt this immense sense of liberation. For the first time in a long while, I began to see a future, one I had dreamed about while I was dying, while I was fighting so hard not to.

The next step was meeting with Dr. Hamid and Nurse Maggie at the Angeles Clinic. The team there had taken a chance on me, offering experimental biochemotherapy as an option to save my life. And I made it! I was told I'd need follow-up treatment, six months of IL-2. Just when I thought I was done with treatments, I was advised to check into the intensive care ward one weekend a month for an IV drip of IL-2. My heart sank. I was 50 pounds lighter, my body completely drained, and I was struggling with brain fog. The thought of more treatment felt unbearable. My mental reserves were completely depleted, and all I wanted was to go back to my life.

There comes a time in a cancer patient's journey when tough decisions have to be made. Some people endure years of chemotherapy, their bodies worn out and fried. Your life becomes reduced to pure survival. I could barely concentrate. I could barely walk two blocks. But I was alive! When it came to continuing the treatments—weekends in a hospital bed being dosed with more poison that had already killed my cancer, I started leaning heavily on the numbers. What were my chances now? I'd started with only a 5% chance of surviving five years. With the ongoing IL-2 treatments, my chances didn't improve. They were about the same as they had been without it. The thought of surviving without more side effects sounded a lot better to me. So, I chose to stop the treatments. Some cancer patients choose to end their treatment, and I completely understand why.

Post Treatment

Obviously, the treatment itself was brutal. I was a shell of a human, so weak that it took me a long time to truly recover. And there were things I would never get back the same.

One of the hardest parts of recovering from this kind of cancer treatment wasn't just about me, but my entire family. My daughter was really in a dark place. Her recovery from depression took years. As I mentioned before, she had started being bullied in middle school right when I was diagnosed with cancer. Allison had gone from living a peaceful, serene life in Bear Valley—laughing, playing in the forest, and having a childhood full of sunshine, camping trips, skiing, and lake swimming. But when she started at Avery Middle School, everything changed. She was thrust into a world with kids who had known each other since kindergarten. Middle school is brutal. Allison became an easy target, a punching bag for many of those kids. That's when she started cutting.

The year before I was diagnosed with cancer, my husband and I hit a really rough patch. Our marriage was on the brink of collapse, almost leading to a divorce or at least a separation. And, of course, this was incredibly hard on Allison. Then, my cancer diagnosis came, and it pushed her even deeper into a dark place, especially with all the hours I was away. We tried to hold onto our cabin in Bear Valley, and Chris worked hard to keep everything together financially. He took a night shift at the local resort. He thought Allison would sleep while he was gone, and when he came home, he'd take her to the school bus and then catch up on sleep. But Allison was still a kid. She spent too much time on the computer, trying to find some comfort in the isolation. One would think that our community would have stepped in and offered to take her in while Chris worked, but that didn't happen.

I ran out of sick leave, and my salary had to cover the cost of the substitute teacher at my school district. Meanwhile, I lay in the hospital, shivering and shaking from the medication, while Chris was dealing with piles of medical bills. Hundreds of thousands of dollars were due. Eventually, the insurance kicked in and covered everything, but just seeing those numbers was overwhelming. We desperately wanted to hold on to our life in Bear Valley, but it became clear that wasn't going to happen.

Immediately after my cancer treatment, we had to move, which meant Allison had to change schools. On top of the trauma of our near separation and divorce and my almost dying, now she had to leave everything behind and start fresh in a new school. She was supposed to go to Bret Hart High School, but moving to Markleeville, California, meant she would attend school in Gardnerville, Nevada, where ninth grade was still part of middle school. This was disastrous for her mental health. Instead of starting high school with her friends, Allison was thrown into yet another new school. The depression took over, and a dark cloud hovered over her. In the fall of 2011, we received a phone call from the sheriff's department in Douglas County, Nevada. They had taken custody of Allison to keep her safe from herself and from the threats she had written down. To say we were heartbroken is an understatement. Allison was soon committed to West Hills Hospital in Reno, Nevada, where she would spend the month of November.

Allison was completely consumed by massive depression, and we found out she had suicidal ideation. It was unbelievable. Just after I had nearly died, now we were facing this. We had no choice but to keep her in the hospital until the doctors determined she was no longer a threat to her own safety. When she came home, the reality set in. We had to remove all the knives, and anything that could be used to hurt her, like ropes, had to be hidden.

After talking with Allison, I believe the depression was there even before I was diagnosed with cancer. But my diagnosis only deepened the darkness inside of her. The cancer diagnosis seemed to amplify those dark clouds in her mind, clouds that kept her from seeing any kind of future or hope. It made her feel like that was the only way out. The weight of it all was unbearable for her.

Our family became involved in suicide prevention efforts in Gardnerville, Nevada, where Allison attended school, not far from our new home in Markleeville, California. Allison eventually found a therapist, someone who helped her through the darkest times and supported her in finishing high school. There were days when I would check on her constantly, just to make sure she was OK, to make sure she was still alive in her bedroom. If I could've been diagnosed with cancer again to prevent her from going through all that pain and sadness, I would've done it without hesitation. But we all have our emotional battles to face.

I'm happy to report that Allison is now the mother of my granddaughter, Ellie. She's attending college in Oregon to become an ASL interpreter. While life isn't always easy, Allison has more good days now. The sad days of depression lingered for a long time. She's an awesome parent to Ellie!

Chris was traumatized by picking up the mail for years after my treatment. The big, thick envelopes full of hospital bills were a constant reminder of the financial burden we were under. Hundreds of thousands of dollars were due, and I honestly don't know how he held it all together. On top of everything else, he worked nights just to make the payments and keep our cabin in Bear Valley. We loved that cabin so much. But, because we had to move when the school in Bear Valley closed down while I was sick, I wasn't there to defend myself professionally. A group of parents who didn't even like the teachers decided the school wasn't worth keeping open. And here I was, lying in bed, just trying to survive, and I was told that our precious little mountain school was closing. The ripple effects from that moment on were immeasurable. The move, the depression, the loss of our beloved cabin, and the professional setbacks I faced—everything just spiraled out of control as I was thrust into a new work environment, trying to pick up the pieces.

Chris did everything he could to try to save our cabin, but honestly, he could've just given up and let us go into foreclosure sooner if we'd known we'd never be able to stay there. When one person has to leave home to save their life, it puts so much pressure on the other person trying to hold it all together. Not everyone has to leave their home like I did. Some people manage to stay local while going through cancer treatments, but we didn't have that option.

Chris did his best to call me often while I was in the hospital. He knew hearing his and Allison's voices, meant the world to me. But with the medication, I could barely respond to most calls. Still, he'd tell me about the massive snowfall and how the cabin was buried under feet of snow. He'd describe how our neighbor, Jason, would use his snowcat to push the snow away from the house to keep it from collapsing. He'd also talk about how long it took him to drive Allison to the bus stop, how it sometimes took hours to get down the mountain through the snow. It was a huge ordeal, but we loved our life in Bear Valley.

And as I lay in that hospital bed, fighting just to stay alive, I held onto the hope that I would one day return there. Even with everything going on—my illness, the community's efforts to close the school, everything—I dreamed of going back, of somehow making things better. I imagined how I could return and create a special place for kids to learn. Those dreams about the future, about going back to the life we loved, gave me the strength to keep going.

When I returned to the cabin in 2011 after surgery, I was so happy to be home. I remember taking a walk into town and realizing I didn't have the energy to make it back up the hill to our little cabin. I ran into people I knew, but they didn't recognize me because of the physical changes from the cancer treatment. I sat in the cabin, waiting, but no one came by to check in on me, just like when no one checked on my daughter when she was alone while Chris was working. The most beautiful place can be the loneliest places to live. They can be the most unfriendly places to live.

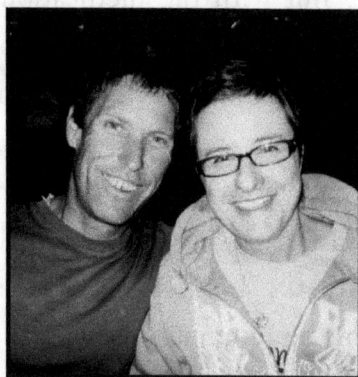

Right after cancer summer 2011

The trifecta I spoke about earlier—the three things that make life manageable—was thrown off balance by the loneliness and unfriendliness of the Bear Valley community. The constant criticism I faced as a teacher in that town created so much stress. I never felt truly welcomed or supported there. I think the isolation and pressure, in combination with the emotional toll of the environment, may have contributed to my cancer.

By August 2011, I was barely hanging on, but I had to return to work. I needed my health insurance to survive. I moved to Markleeville, California, to stay within the Alpine County School District. No one at my school district said, "Take the time you need to heal." I was pushed into returning to work, and my school was closed. The thought of leaving my cabin, of uprooting my entire family again, felt heartless. We moved to a new town just to keep my insurance and survive, but in the process, I was made to feel like I was being pushed out of the school district. Later, I learned the administration had been overheard saying that I wouldn't make the move because I was too sick. It was gut-wrenching to hear that. The heartless things people say and do when you're fighting for your life are unbelievable. Cancer patients need support.

Despite everything, my family persevered. We did our best to make things work when Allison returned after her treatment for depression, trying to heal together. But deep down, we knew the cancer could come back and that I only had a 5% chance of surviving five years. Our finances were in ruins, with no savings left; moving had drained everything. We were left with a huge stack of bills we couldn't pay. We tried renting out our cabin, but eventually, it went into foreclosure, and losing it broke our hearts.

During this time, I began painting. I painted angels. I felt like they were a part of my survival. At first, they were just outlines of little bird-like creatures, which later turned into more childlike images. I taught myself how to paint, and it brought me comfort as we tried to adjust to our new community. My new school wasn't always friendly, but there were people there who would become lifelong friends. Allison met the man she would marry at her new school, and Chris found his place at a new ski area. The Bowens were doing everything we could to get back to the mountain life we loved.

Physically, I started getting stronger. For the first three years after treatment, I was still very thin, and my hair grew back short and curly, like a little baby's. Chemo brain was real, though, and I struggled with remembering my new students' names and grading third-grade math papers. On top of that, I continued to face mistreatment from a bullying administrator at my school district. Nobody thought I'd actually make a move, but there I was, pushing through each day to keep a paycheck and health insurance. I had been the main breadwinner for our family as a school teacher for years, and without that job, we didn't know what we would do. I needed health insurance for my check-ups to make sure the cancer was still gone.

Even though the school administration kept trying to get rid of me, the community was incredibly welcoming. I met so many kind people who couldn't believe I was walking after everything I had been through. Allison started making friends at her new school - some of whom stayed with her into adulthood, while others have drifted away. We did our best to focus on the things that brought us happiness despite the constant cancer check-ups.

Realizing that Los Angeles was too far for the check-ups I needed to survive, we went to Stanford in California. I was a patient there for about two years until I found a doctor in Carson Valley, Nevada. That's when I understood there were different levels of cancer care. Fortunately, Dr. Kelley at the Carson Valley Cancer Center was honest enough to admit that he might not have all the answers for me, but he could order my PET scans and check to see if I was still NED (No Evidence of Disease).

Physically, my body constantly hurt. I could barely make it through a full day of school, often leaving early just to sit in a recliner and cry. The side effects of chemotherapy and immunotherapy had destroyed my joints, and I was in constant pain. When I was assigned to teach kindergarten, it was a real struggle because of how much time I had to spend squatting down next to kids or sitting on the rug with them. Everything inside me hurt. Over time, my cognitive abilities started to improve. Finding joy in the small things and leaning on my angels helped me get through. I would dive into painting, letting my senses guide me. If my angel

95

wanted to be red to represent a fighting spirit, I'd paint it red. If it felt like purple, I'd make it purple. Day by day, we made it through.

About three years after treatment, I was getting better at remembering names. Allison was still frustrated with me, though, as I would forget so many things. The good news was that I got back on my skis! My family and I would ski at Kirkwood, near Lake Tahoe, California. Our love for the outdoors really kept us going. Being in nature was always so healing. My personal trifecta was starting to improve: the community was warm and welcoming, and the place where we lived was beautiful. But, unfortunately, my work environment was still toxic.

When a school district wants to get rid of a tenured teacher, they start bullying them, giving them terrible assignments, changing grade levels every year, and micromanaging everything they do, as if they don't know what they're doing. All of this was happening to me, and I realized I couldn't come home crying every day. It was really bad for my health. It became clear that it was time for us to move somewhere new, so I started looking at areas in California where we could start fresh.

I hit a major milestone in surviving cancer - five years! It was a huge moment for me. I knew it was time to take control and create a future for myself and my family, one that left fear behind. I needed to stop being stressed and feeling harassed. So, Chris and I decided to move to Groveland, California, where I got hired at another small mountain school. My career didn't get any easier, though. I worked another six years as a public school teacher. Eventually, early "retirement" became necessary because the job just wasn't sustainable mentally. Beating cancer gave me the courage to stay true to myself. I wasn't going to settle anymore.

My cancer checkups would take me back to Los Angeles to resume with Dr. Hamid. I didn't trust anyone else. It was important for me to go to the place that had saved my life. I traveled there for PET scans, CT scans, and blood work at the Angeles Clinic. Each time, I was told I was NED - cancer-free! Over time, my anxiety about these tests lessened. Now, I have virtually no worry about cancer coming back. After 14 years, Dr. Hamid told me he considers me cured.

How has being a survivor influenced my life? I feel like every day is a miracle. My decisions today reflect what is best for me. I have survived and beaten the odds.

Survivor's guilt is real. For a long time, I felt a deep sadness every time I heard about a "melahomie," the term the melanoma community uses for each other, passing away. There was the sweet young woman I met by chance in Gardnerville, Nevada, who had been experiencing back pain that turned out to be late-stage melanoma. She passed away about six months after being diagnosed. There was the handsome young father in Santa Cruz who lost his battle with ocular melanoma, leaving behind a young daughter and wife. A very sick young woman I met at a melanoma walk passed away not long after. There were so many encounters with cancer patients who are no longer here, and each one left a mark on my heart.

Why? Why did I survive such a terrible diagnosis while others didn't? These melahomies were younger than me when they died. I couldn't understand why I made it through. My life after cancer treatment has been about mentally facing survival - trying to process why I was the one to survive when so many others didn't.

I took that guilt and transformed it into action. My goal became to educate others about the dangers of skin cancer. So many people think it's something you can "just cut out," not realizing it can metastasize into something deadly. I started a blog to raise awareness. Back in the early 2010s, blogs were a powerful way to educate, inform, and share ideas.

I found myself at a 5K fundraiser walk/run in Alameda, California, for Aim at Melanoma. I loved the organization's mission and its grassroots beginnings. It sparked a passion in me to raise funds for Aim, so I started coordinating my own walks. That's when I truly connected with the melanoma community. Through these events, I was able to raise money for research in hopes of finding a cure. It always felt incredible to finish a fundraiser and see how much we could accomplish. These events gave people a space to honor their loved ones who had passed from melanoma, while also raising awareness for those who happened to stumble upon our cause.

But, inevitably, there were always melanoma patients at the event who didn't make it to the next year. People died, and that sadness only fueled my drive to do more. Then, the pandemic hit, and it changed the landscape for these types of fundraisers. It became difficult to recreate the success of the walks I had hosted before Covid, but I kept trying, knowing how much those events meant to the community.

The most amazing moments I experienced after surviving cancer were the family milestones. I made it to Allison's 8th grade graduation, her high school graduation, her wedding, and the birth of my granddaughter, Ellie. Being a grandma is hands down the best reward for beating cancer 14 years ago.

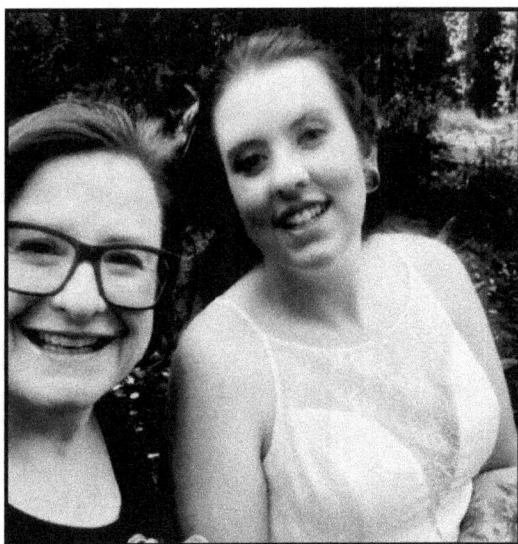

I decided to quit teaching full-time—it was just too stressful. I still work, but I've shifted to jobs that are less demanding than education. Travel has become a huge part of my life. Since beating cancer, I've been to Costa Rica with Allison, hiked Hadrian's Wall in Northern England, and tackled the Heiz-Hexen Steig Trail in Northern Germany. I'm planning an adventure in the Patagonia region of South America next. Life is for adventures! My cancer check-ups have simplified. Now it's just blood tests. No more PET scans or brain MRIs. The dermatologist is still an annual appointment, but these visits no longer bring me anxiety.

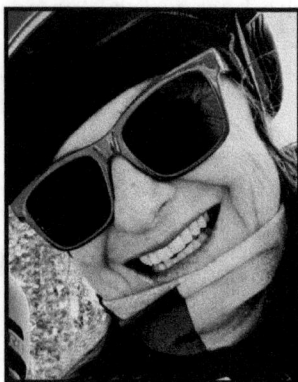

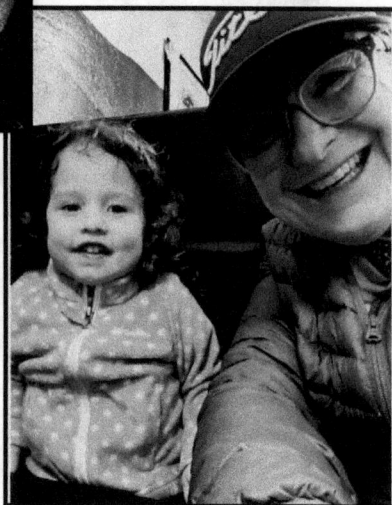

I still have a deep passion for cancer awareness and advocacy. Writing this allows me to scratch that itch and share my message. It's so important for people to know that there is hope even when things look darkest. Even with a late-stage diagnosis, there is hope. Many of us have beaten the odds.

Getting a cancer diagnosis completely overwhelms your senses. You're hit with a million questions. What are my odds of survival? Will I need chemo? Will I lose my hair? Family members start wondering how much time they have left with you. The trauma of living through cancer is real, and it doesn't just affect the person diagnosed; it changes everyone involved.

Surviving

There are many emotions when you survive late-stage cancer, especially when you are given only a 5% chance of living five years. It was a roller coaster just to not die. The first four years after treatment were filled with so many emotions. It was almost like coming back from a war. I wanted to tell everyone what had happened to me.

The after-effects of survival are the following:

- Depression: I found out that interferon causes depression. I could not stop randomly crying. Tears rolled down my face quite frequently and I thought the cancer would return, it was only a matter of time.
- Fatigue and Body Aches: I experienced extreme fatigue for years. I don't even know how I made it through a day of teaching. My body hurt so much that when I was given a teaching assignment for preschool students, simply getting up off the ground hurt. The treatment caused me to have arthritic conditions. Exhaustion was normal.

- Brain Fog: I had to use a teacher's edition textbook to grade 3rd-grade math. My brain functioning was not ok. Being in a new school meant learning new student's names. Chemo-brain is real. My daughter would become frustrated with me when I did not remember her friends' names.

Present

Now that it's been 14 years since I fought cancer, I look back in amazement that this is actually my story, that I made it through an unimaginable diagnosis. Today, I live with a deep desire to make every moment count. I know I'm on borrowed time, and that thought stays with me. Life is truly precious, and I don't take it for granted. My decisions now are all about having as many adventures as I can! I've traveled to Costa Rica to see sloths, hiked the stunning green countryside and Hadrian's Wall in England, and explored the Harz-Hexenstieg Trail in Germany. Skiing in Argentina is next on the list for another trekking adventure. Being alive is a gift, and I plan to live every moment true to my heart.

I would want others to know - don't wait for a cancer diagnosis to start being true to yourself. When you're faced with death, all you have left are your memories to carry you through. And for me, those memories will be of the adventures I've had. I want people to remember me as someone who took chances, someone who lived fully and thought, Steph sure had a lot of adventures! And, of course, I'm excited to teach my granddaughter how to ski.

Advice

Advice for the newly diagnosed:

- Allow yourself all the feelings! You will be angry, you will be sad, and you will be scared. Hearing the words that you have cancer shocks the system. Allow yourself to cry. A flood of emotions will cascade through your brain and it will take mental strength to step into your new role as a cancer patient.
- Gather a team: your family and friends. You will want someone to attend doctor appointments with you and drive you. You will want someone to take notes and ask questions. Allow people to help you!
- Be okay with not understanding everything your doctor says. Take time to research the treatment options and do what is best for you. Listening to the medical terminology can be confusing and it takes time to sort through the information.

- Find an online support group of others who have experienced a similar diagnosis. The emotional support from others helps keep your spirits lifted!
- If you do not feel as if your doctor is really rooting for you and has your back, get a second opinion. Do not worry about hurting someone's feelings, doctors are people and some are more knowledgeable than others. Do what is best for you!
- Use online resources, like Aim at Melanoma or the Melanoma Research Foundation for updated information. Both of these organizations advocate for advancements in treatment and information for patients.

Call to Action

It is time for people to know just how dangerous melanoma skin cancer can be. It has had a reputation of being something "you can just cut out" but it is so much more complicated. People who have experienced melanoma cannot be on any organ donation programs. Did you know that we cannot give blood? Melanoma is known as the black beast and it is an insidious illness that, like in my case, hid for a decade before coming back as stage four. Many people do not know where their melanoma originated as it simply appears internally as a stage four cancer. Melanoma cancer can be prevented if caught early and is one of the most preventable cancers when people take precautions while out in the sun. Supporting melanoma awareness is saving lives.

www.ingramcontent.com/pod-product-compliance
Lightning Source LLC
Chambersburg PA
CBHW070810280326
41934CB00012B/3140